The Clean Eating
SLOW COOKER

A Healthy Cookbook of Wholesome Meals that Prep Fast and Cook Slow

LINDA LARSEN

Foreword by Sonja Overhiser, *A Couple Cooks*

ROCKRIDGE
PRESS

I dedicate this book to my dear husband, Doug; my beautiful nieces Maddie and Grace; and my wonderful nephew Michael. They are a joy and a delight!

For general information on our other products and services or to obtain technical support, please contact our Customer Care Department within the United States at (866) 744-2665, or outside the United States at (510) 253-0500.

Rockridge Press publishes its books in a variety of electronic and print formats. Some content that appears in print may not be available in electronic books, and vice versa.

Design by Anne Kenady

Photography © Suzanne Clements/Stocksy, cover; Nadianb/Shutterstock, cover (background); Victoria Firmston/Stockfood, p. 4; Gareth Morgans/Stockfood, p. 10; Gallo Images Pty Ltd./Stockfood, p. 24; Susan Brooks-Dammann/Stocksy, p. 34; Great Stock!/Stockfood, p. 46 and back cover; Natasa Mandic/Stocksy, p. 64 and back cover; Tanya Zouev/Stockfood, p. 82; Louise Lister/Stockfood, p. 100; Hein van Tonder/Stockfood, p. 120; Great Stock!/Stockfood, p. 138; Jonathan Gregson/Stockfood, p. 156 and back cover; Catja Vedder/Stockfood, p. 172.

ISBN Print 978-1-62315-910-8 | eBook 978-1-62315-911-5

THE CLEAN EATING SLOW COOKER

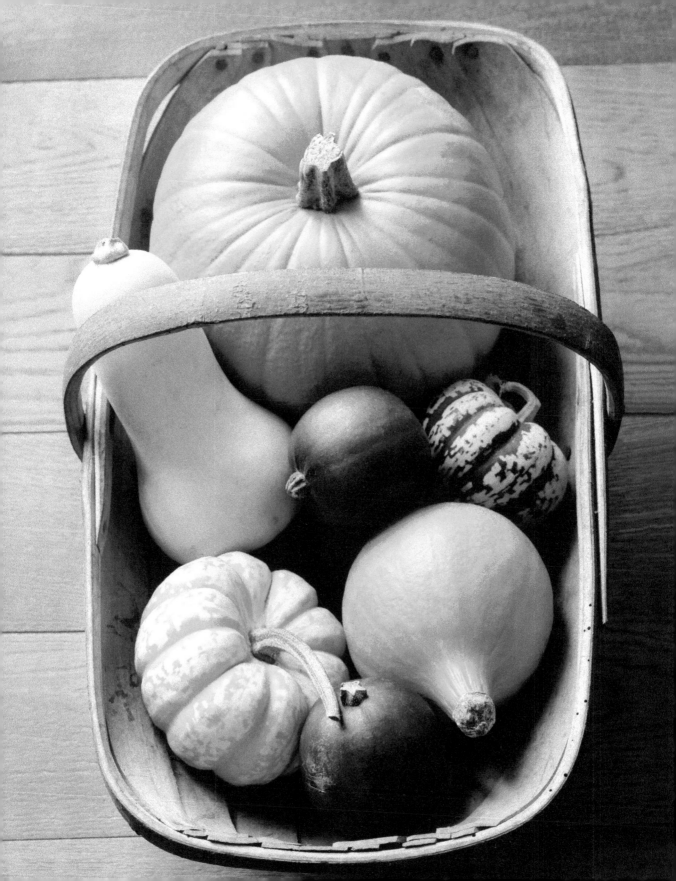

contents

foreword

If you had told me ten years ago I'd be writing the foreword to a healthy cookbook, I'd have thought you were pulling my leg. At that time, what I considered "cooking" was toaster pastries and breakfast cereal. Recently married, my husband Alex and I ate whatever was quickest, like fast food Mexican and frozen pizzas. I didn't even know how to boil water for pasta.

Fast-forward ten years, and our lives have shifted drastically. It certainly didn't happen overnight, but little by little, real, unprocessed whole food started to creep in. I ate at my first farm-to-table restaurant and tasted flavors I never knew existed. Friends made us homemade dinners of sushi and cheese soufflé and pasta puttanesca. We discovered Julia Child and her passion for honest home cooking. We bought eggs at the farmers' market from a farmer who knew our names. We started growing herbs in little pots on our front steps. We tossed out the old salad dressings in our refrigerator and began whisking our own vinaigrettes.

Somewhere along the way, good, clean food became our norm, and our lives have never been better. We have more energy, fewer stomachaches, and we're a whole lot happier. People started to ask us how we did it, so we created a website to share our recipes. It's now grown to national acclaim, and our first cookbook of whole-food vegetarian recipes is set to publish in early 2018.

In a perfect world, the transition to eating clean would be as easy as 1, 2, 3. But it's not so simple. While healthy cooking can be incredibly fun-filled and joyful, it also takes time and effort. Locating recipes, sourcing ingredients, finding the time and space for it all—these are major barriers for today's home cook. We're all busy. We need a quick, reliable way to put healthy food on the table.

Enter the slow cooker. Slow cooking is so hassle-free, it's easier to fit cooking into your everyday routine. And while past generations used slow cookers to cook high-fat, processed foods, Linda Larsen is here to show you a better way.

Linda's story is similar to ours. In 2010, she started to make a transition from sugary treats to good, clean food. In *The Clean Eating Slow Cooker*, she has created the best and only guide to eating clean with all the time-saving and nutrient-preserving advantages of a slow cooker. Her healthy foods become even more delicious after several hours of long, slow heat. Think Pumpkin Pie Baked Oatmeal, Eggplant Parmesan, Shrimp and Grits, and Spinach and Artichoke Dip—all made of whole-food ingredients and slow-cooked to perfection.

Ten years ago I wouldn't have believed it.

—Sonja Overhiser, *A Couple Cooks*

introduction

I have a confession to make: I used to absolutely adore sugar. I simply loved eating anything made with chocolate; my favorite treat was peanut butter cups. I considered a meal something to get through before I could have dessert. But about 10 years ago I realized that I was not doing myself any favors by treating my body this way. I found the concept of eating clean.

Eating clean is a concept that began in the 1970s and really took off in America about 10 years ago when Tosca Reno introduced the plan in her popular books. The concept is simple, but in this day of the frozen dinners and microwave popcorn, it may seem too simple. All you have to do is eat lower on the food chain. Instead of an apple turnover, eat an apple. Instead of buying a can of (sodium laden) soup, make your own. Shop around the edges of the grocery store and don't buy any food that contains more than a few ingredients. Eating this way will help you slim down, give you more energy, lower your risk of illness, and save you money! What could be better?

Well, I know what you're thinking: This sounds like a lot more work. And cooking from scratch is more difficult and time-consuming than microwaving a TV dinner. But the payoff is tremendous, in terms of better health, more energy, and a fatter wallet. And there is one way to make eating clean much simpler.

Add a slow cooker to your eating clean plan! The slow cooker makes it so easy to eat clean. For most of these recipes, you do a little chopping and slicing, fill up the slow cooker, and let the appliance do the rest of the work. You'll come home to dinner already prepared, with the house smelling so good you'll wonder why you ever stopped for fast food on the way home in the bad old days. And cleanup is easy too; just clean the slow cooker insert and you're done!

Now, this may all sound too simple. I know there are days when that peanut butter cup sounds so good, or perhaps your coworker brought her famous double fudge coconut brownies for a midafternoon treat. One of the best things about the clean eating plan is that you don't have to slavishly stick to your diet. Most people do best when their diet is about 80 to 90 percent clean, which allows for some treats. That doesn't mean you can completely fall off the wagon. But knowing that you can occasionally have a slice of lemon cake will help you stick to the eating clean plan.

In this book you'll find delicious (and easy) recipes for everything from snacks to main dishes, from soups to vegetables. Almost all use ten ingredients or fewer, all take less than 20 minutes prep time or less, and all use whole, nutritious foods. Every recipe contains nutrition information so you can see that they are healthy.

After a few weeks of eating clean, you'll notice some changes. Your skin will be clearer. Your hair will be shinier. You will have more energy. You will probably lose some weight. You'll notice you are spending less money on food. And you will feel good, too, which is the best motivator for sticking with a lifestyle change.

Because that's what eating clean is. It's not a diet. It's not a fad. It's a way of feeding yourself and taking care of yourself and your family that you can live with for life. Once you understand the concepts of eating clean and slow cooking, you can branch out and create your own favorite recipes just by tweaking some of the choices in this book. And you'll never look back. Let's get started!

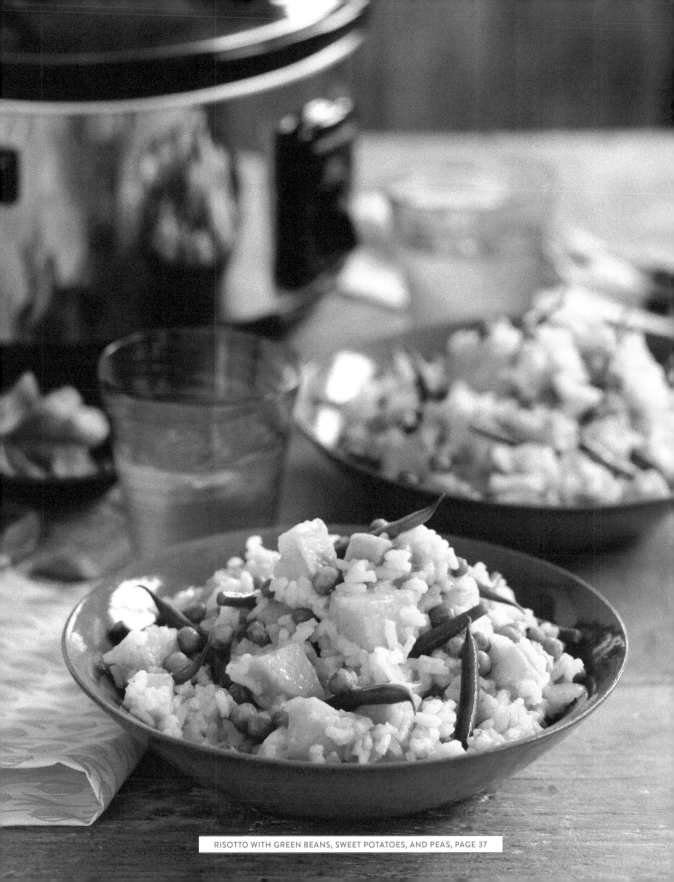

RISOTTO WITH GREEN BEANS, SWEET POTATOES, AND PEAS, PAGE 37

CHAPTER ONE

CLEAN AND SLOW

The concepts in this book, clean eating and slow cooking, are natural partners. The slow cooker is designed to cook whole foods in the healthiest way possible, with low and slow heat. Soups, stews, casseroles, breakfasts, side dishes, and desserts are almost effortless to make. And everything tastes so fresh and good!

Why We Eat Clean

Did you know that the average American eats about 7 pounds of food additives a year? Those ingredients include artificial colors, artificial flavors, nitrates, preservatives, emulsifiers, stabilizers, gums, MSG, high-fructose corn syrup, and trans fat. And those compounds do nothing to promote health; they are all added by the food industry to get you to crave fake foods and to make them more money.

To get an idea of what you are really eating when you buy processed foods, take a look at a food label the next time you shop. The ingredients in a frozen chicken pot pie can include cellulose gum, BHA, BHT, corn syrup solids, lard, carrageenan, MSG, mechanically separated chicken, sodium stearoyl lactylate, and hydrogenated fats. You would not include any of those ingredients in your own homemade pot pie! And the nutrition numbers for that food are even scarier. One serving of a frozen pot pie can contain 1,000 mg of sodium, get 50 percent of the calories from fat, and contain 15 grams of saturated fat.

These ingredients not only do nothing for your health, but they can actually cause addiction as well. Many food companies add lots of fat, sugar, and salt to the "foods" they produce so you will buy more. Studies have shown that addiction to sugar and fat, for instance, can be as serious and as difficult to kick as an addiction to heroin!

So what's a nutrition-conscious person to do? Believe it or not, there is a simple solution. Eat clean. Stop buying (most) foods with a label. Avoid the frozen food section of the grocery store, with one exception: You can buy plain frozen vegetables and fruits with nothing added. And shop mainly around the outside aisles of the grocery store. Those inside aisles are where all the processed foods lurk.

The five primary benefits of clean eating include better health, more energy, a reduced risk of developing diseases, spending less money at the grocery store (and at restaurants), and not feeling hungry. Your health will improve because you are no longer eating fat-, additive-, and sodium-laden processed foods; you will probably lose weight too. You'll have more energy because your body will be properly fueled and can move like it is supposed to. Many of the diseases that plague our modern life are associated with a poor diet; your risk for those illnesses will decrease when you eat clean. And your pocketbook will be fatter because the clean foods you'll buy cost less than processed foods!

The Five Pillars of Clean Eating

There are five pillars of clean eating that guide every choice you will make as you shop and cook. They include choosing whole unprocessed foods, avoiding processed foods, eating frequent small meals, combining proteins and carbohydrates at every meal, and cooking your own meals. Let's go through each in some detail.

1. CHOOSING WHOLE UNPROCESSED FOODS

Whole foods are the lowest foods on the food chain. That means you will buy whole apples, carrots, lean meats, whole-grain pasta, dairy products, and other simple foods. These are foods that are minimally processed. In other words, they are foods that your great-grandmother would recognize. These foods have the ideal combinations of protein, fat, sugars, vitamins, and minerals that your body needs. And they also contain micronutrients that you just can't get from boxed mac and cheese mix or frozen pizza. Or a vitamin pill.

2. AVOIDING PROCESSED FOODS

Processed foods have labels, and those labels can contain long lists of strange sounding ingredients. If you try to avoid buying foods with a label, you'll have an easier time abiding by this pillar. You can buy some processed foods: canned tomato puree in BPA-free cans, whole-grain pasta, or any food that has fewer than five ingredients. But don't buy any food that contains an ingredient you can't pronounce. If you wouldn't add disodium inosinate to your homemade pasta sauce, don't put it into your body!

3. EATING FREQUENT SMALL MEALS

Eating frequent small meals is one of the best perks of the eating clean lifestyle. Eat a good breakfast, lunch, and dinner, and have two snacks during the day. This pillar ensures that you will not be hungry and won't be tempted by that chocolate-frosted doughnut during a break at work. Eating frequently also boosts your metabolism and helps keep your blood glucose steady throughout the day so you have lots of energy.

4. COMBINING PROTEINS AND CARBOHYDRATES AT EVERY MEAL

Every meal or snack should combine protein and carbohydrates because this will help you feel full. Eating a banana by itself is good, but think about pairing that banana with some almond butter instead. This combination will also help you avoid cravings for sugar and fat.

5. COOKING YOUR OWN MEALS

And the last pillar of the clean eating lifestyle is cooking your own meals. If you aren't an experienced cook, this can seem daunting. But that's where this book will help! Buy a good slow cooker and try some of these recipes. You'll quickly learn your way around the kitchen. Before you know it, you'll be making homemade bread, eating delicious meals you made yourself, and feeling great.

ON THE EDGE

There are some foods you want to avoid while you are eating clean. Don't buy these five food products (I can't call them foods) when you're at the store.

1. **Condiments** can be problematic. Commercially produced mayonnaise, salad dressings, and mustard are usually loaded with salt and can contain emulsifiers and stabilizers. Read labels carefully if you choose to use these ingredients or make your own.

2. **Margarines, spreadable butters, and other spreads** have lots of fake ingredients and should be avoided. Many are made with hydrogenated shortening that contains trans fats, the most dangerous type of fat. Trans fats become part of your body's cells, weakening their structure and function. These products also contain artificial colors and other additives.

3. **Artificial sweeteners** fool your body into thinking you are eating something sweet. Your brain then releases a compound that activates the pleasure center of your brain. But when no calories follow, your body becomes confused and you will crave more food. This can lead to weight gain, can be addictive, and can even change the way you taste foods. People who consume very intense fake sweeteners can start to crave more sweets.

4. **Microwave popcorn** is a real convenience, and popcorn makes a great snack. But the processed products can be made with GMO corn, and there are lots of weird chemicals in the bag. One compound in particular, perfluorooctanoic acid, is linked to infertility and liver cancer. Pop your own popcorn on the stove.

5. **Farmed-raised salmon** can be high in compounds such as PCBs, dioxin, and DDT—chemicals that are linked to cancer. Wild-caught Alaska salmon is your best bet. It is a great source of omega-3 fatty acids, protein, and B vitamins.

Is It Clean?

So what is considered "clean" in the food world? A clean food is minimally processed or not processed at all. Corn on the cob is clean; frozen corn in butter sauce is not. A grilled lean steak is clean; Chinese Pepper Steak from the local takeout place is not.

These are the foods you should choose as you embark on the eating clean lifestyle.

FRUITS: Most fruits are on the eating clean plan. Choose fresh apples, bananas, strawberries, raspberries, peaches, plums, melons, oranges, grapefruit, lemons, papayas, mangoes, and cherries. You can buy frozen fruits too, but make sure they don't have any added sugar. Canned fruits can be eaten on this plan, but again, make sure no sugar is added, whether it's regular sugar or corn syrup, and the cans are BPA-free. BPA is a chemical used to make plastic can liners and may have an effect on the brain and behavior. Dried fruits are also good, as long as they are made without sugar.

VEGETABLES: Load up on vegetables! These wonderful foods are packed full of micronutrients that can help prevent illness. Buy broccoli, cauliflower, kale and other leafy greens, tomatoes, celery, bell peppers, asparagus, avocado, potatoes, sweet potatoes, carrots, parsnips, onions, cucumbers, garlic, squash, and zucchini. If you buy frozen vegetables, make sure that the only ingredient is that vegetable. Canned vegetables should be purchased only if they are in BPA-free cans.

MEATS: Lean meats are a cornerstone of the eating clean plan. Choose lean cuts of beef such as London broil, top round, sirloin tip, sirloin steak, strip steak, and lean hamburger.

POULTRY AND FISH: Poultry is a great choice for eating clean. Choose chicken breasts, whole chickens, ground chicken, turkey tenderloin, ground turkey breast, and chicken thighs. Remove the skin from chicken and turkey before you cook it, for less fat. Fish is a great choice too; choose white fish fillets such as halibut and mahi mahi, salmon fillets and steaks, and shellfish such as scallops. Remember that swordfish and tuna can be high in mercury.

COCONUT OIL

Coconut oil is used frequently in clean cooking for several reasons. Many people think this fat is unhealthy because it contains saturated fat, but recent research has shown that saturated fat is not as bad for you as previously thought. And coconut oil is mostly made up of medium chain fatty acids (MCFAs). That type of fat is not easily stored in the body, has antimicrobial properties, and is easier to digest.

As long as you buy organic, virgin coconut oil, you are getting great health benefits. MCFAs are immediately processed by your liver, which means your body uses them as energy instead of storing them as fat. Coconut oil has high levels of antioxidants, which help reduce inflammation in the body. The lauric acid in coconut oil turns into a compound called monolaurin when it is digested. That compound kills the yeast *Candida albicans* and also kills *Staphylococcus aureus*.

In studies, coconut oil reduced total and LDL cholesterol in the blood (the bad kind) and increased HDL cholesterol (the good kind). This can help protect you against heart disease.

And coconut oil does not make food taste like coconut! The flavor is very mild, and you won't even notice it in the foods you cook.

GRAINS, BEANS, AND NUTS: Whole grains, beans, and nuts have a definite place on the eating clean plan. Barley, millet, oats, whole-wheat pasta, farro, wild rice, brown rice, and quinoa are delicious in salads and soups. Also choose kidney beans, lentils, black beans, pinto beans, and cannellini beans, whether dried or canned, for fiber and phytonutrients. Choose walnuts, cashews, almonds, and peanuts for snacks and to add texture to baked goods.

DAIRY: Low-fat dairy is a good addition to the eating clean lifestyle. Greek yogurt, cottage cheese, low-fat milk, and cheeses provide lots of protein and vitamin D. You can drink almond or rice milk in place of cow's milk.

Slow and Steady

If you have never used a slow cooker before, you are in for a treat. I consider this appliance an essential kitchen component. In fact, it's almost like having your own chef! It's so easy to use; in most recipes, once the food is in the slow cooker, you can just forget about it until it's time to eat. Because you usually don't have to stir the food or check on it while it's cooking, the slow cooker saves time and effort. Since many recipes call for you to sauté something, then turn it or stir it, add something else, then assemble it, and bake it in the oven, many people just don't bother. But the one-step cooking process of the slow cooker couldn't be easier.

And there are other benefits to using a slow cooker. First, the low temperature prevents harmful compounds from forming as the food cooks. Compounds called advanced glycation end products (AGEs) can form in food when proteins and fat are heated at high temperatures, such as when you grill a steak. These compounds cause inflammation and stress to the cells in your body. In fact, AGEs are linked to the development of diabetes, may harm your kidneys, and may speed up the aging process. But the low temperature of the slow cooker (about 180°F on low and about 230°F on high) prevents these compounds from forming.

And this low cooking temperature may also make the food more nutritious. Very high heat destroys vitamin C, so more of this vitamin will be in slow-cooked foods. And many nutrients are water-soluble, which means they will escape the food through steam. Since the slow cooker lid forms a seal, keeping steam inside the appliance, these nutrients will stay in the food.

Slow cooking is simple and wholesome. In fact, it's similar to a pot of soup your grandmother kept simmering on the back burner of her stove. Clean eating is a return to simpler, healthier food. The slow cooker complements the eating clean lifestyle because of its simplicity.

SLOW-COOKING STANDOUTS

Some foods are naturally suited to the slow cooker's long, slow, moist cooking time. Many of the recipes in this book use these ingredients.

Root vegetables are ideal for the slow cooker. Carrots, potatoes, sweet potatoes, parsnips, celery root, and turnips contain lots of fiber and many vitamins and minerals. They cook to tender perfection in the slow cooker.

Lean meats cook beautifully in the slow cooker. In fact, fatty meats and the more expensive beef cuts, such as filet mignon, are not recommended for this appliance. The long, slow cooking time helps break down the fibers and connective tissue in cheaper cuts of beef and pork. That tissue melts, adding flavor to the meat and making it fork tender. And because these leaner meats are cheaper, they save money too.

Dried beans and legumes are perfect for the slow cooker. These foods are very high in fiber, nutrients, protein, and antioxidants, which may help prevent the risk of cancer. They are also inexpensive. A 1-pound bag of black beans, for instance, can feed eight people and costs less than $1.

Chicken thighs are perfect for the slow cooker. White meat can overcook fairly quickly and become tough and dry. But the extra fat in chicken thighs protects them from the long cooking time. This ingredient is cheaper than chicken breasts as well.

Wild rice is one of my favorite slow cooker ingredients. This rice (it's technically a grass seed) is nutty and chewy when perfectly cooked. The slow cooker makes the perfect wild rice every time.

The Slow Cooker Household

Using a slow cooker may be easy, but you still need to plan your meals and think about how you shop and cook.

If the slow cooker is going to be the main appliance you use, you may want to buy more than one. Slow cookers are inexpensive; the most costly is usually around $100. I also like to have two slow cookers of different sizes depending on what I want to cook.

The most important tip for eating clean with your slow cooker is to plan your meals for the week. Look at the foods you have in your pantry, fridge, and freezer. Make a list of what's on hand (and check expiration dates). Then choose the recipes you want to make for the next week.

A shopping list is next. Write down the foods you need to buy to make the recipes you have chosen. Look at the list of the foods you already have in the house to make sure you aren't buying more than you need. Post the recipe list on your refrigerator or pantry door and refer to it to make sure that you stick to the plan.

If you have the storage space, it's a great idea to buy foods that you use often in bulk. Bulk foods are less expensive and may give you more of a choice than buying in smaller quantities. And they use less packaging, especially if you have glass or plastic containers to hold them in your pantry. Dried beans, legumes, rice, pasta, oatmeal, flour, and seeds are all good bulk purchases. But make sure that you will actually use those items before you stock up.

Using leftovers wisely is another smart strategy. Some leftovers, cooked kidney beans, for example, can be used in other recipes such as chili or a casserole. Others will make another meal. Be sure to store leftovers promptly. All leftovers should be refrigerated within 2 hours of cooking time. And don't store foods in the fridge longer than 4 days; freeze them for longer storage.

MORE OR LESS: ADJUST FOR DIFFERENT QUANTITIES

The recipes in this book were developed for a 6-quart slow cooker. That makes enough food to feed six to eight people. Remember that a slow cooker should always be filled at least half full. If there is less food in the appliance, it may overcook and burn. Too much food in the slow cooker means the appliance could overflow or the food will not cook through in the allotted time.

Most of these recipes are very tolerant. That doesn't mean they can take a joke—it means you can adjust the quantities of food and the recipe will still be good. So if you have a 4-quart slow cooker, just reduce all of the quantities in these recipes by about 30 percent. If you have a 7-quart slow cooker, increase the quantities by about 20 percent.

And remember that you don't have to be that precise when you use the slow cooker. For soups, for instance, add enough ingredients and liquid to fill two-thirds of the slow cooker. For a casserole, add more chopped vegetables. If you are making stock, just increase or decrease the amount of water and solids. The recipe will still be wonderful!

Be sure that you write down the correct amounts for your slow cooker, so the next time you make the recipe you won't have to make these calculations again.

Slow Cooker Pro Tips

Once you are used to using the slow cooker, you may want to branch out and create your own recipes. That's fun—as long as you remember that there are some tips to make sure every recipe is delicious and perfectly cooked.

First, many foods should be layered in the slow cooker. The heat at the bottom of the appliance is higher than the heat at the top. Foods that take longer to cook, such as root vegetables and dried beans, should be put into the slow cooker first. Then add other ingredients, such as tender vegetables and meats, on top.

Meats should be thawed before you add them to the slow cooker. There are some recipes out there that call for cooking frozen meats. But if you have someone in your household who is at higher risk for foodborne illness (young children, a pregnant woman, someone with a chronic illness), only use thawed meats in these recipes. Frozen meats may linger in the danger zone of 40°F to 140°F too long when cooked in the slow cooker, and bacteria can grow. The bacteria will be killed when the food temperature reaches 165°F, but those pathogens can produce heat-resistant toxins while they grow that can make someone sick.

If you want to add fresh herbs to your food, add them at the end of cooking time. Long, slow, moist heat tends to leach the flavor out of fresh herbs.

Add dairy products at the end of cooking time. Cheeses, milk, yogurt, and cottage cheese can curdle if cooked for a long period of time.

And to thicken sauces, you can add a slurry of cornstarch or flour mixed with water or broth. Since liquids don't evaporate in the slow cooker, some sauces may be runnier than you prefer. Stir the slurry into the slow cooker and cook on high for another 10 minutes or so until the sauce thickens.

About the Recipes

The recipes in this book were chosen for their use of whole, unprocessed foods; nutrient density; and easy and quick preparation. All of these recipes use fresh, whole foods, with the exception of tomato paste and some canned products.

Each recipe is labeled with a few defining words, including "Dairy-Free," "Gluten-Free," "Nut-Free," and "Vegetarian/Vegan." The recipes with those labels do not contain those ingredients. Vegetarian recipes may contain some cheese or dairy, but vegan recipes have just vegetables, nuts, seeds, and fruit.

Most of the ingredients in these recipes need no preparation other than chopping and peeling. Some meats may be browned before they are added to the slow cooker for added taste and appearance. Ground meats must always be browned first, since they contain more fat and the texture is better if they are cooked first.

No nutrition limits were set for these recipes, although all of the recipes include nutritional information. That's one of the great things about the eating clean plan. You don't have to count fat grams or calories or worry about carbohydrate content. Whole, fresh foods are naturally good for you and provide the right amounts of calories and nutrients your body needs.

The recipes in *The Clean Eating Slow Cooker* require a 6-quart slow cooker, but if the size of your slow cooker is different, remember that you can change the ingredient amounts to suit it.

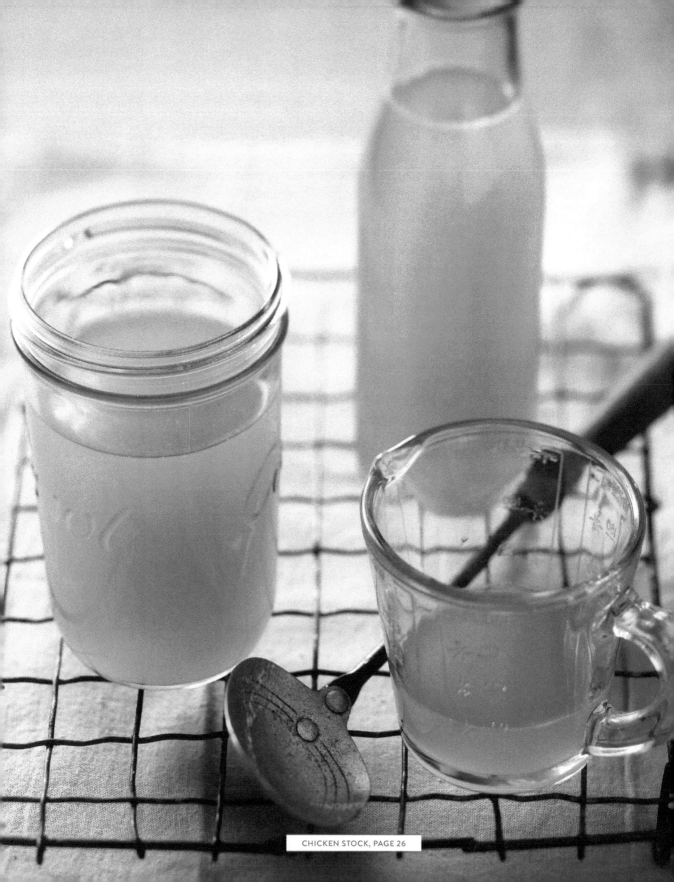

CHICKEN STOCK, PAGE 26

CHAPTER TWO

STOCKS, BROTHS, AND SAUCES

CHICKEN STOCK

MAKES 14 CUPS; SERVING SIZE ½ CUP // PREP TIME: 10 MINUTES
COOK TIME: 7 TO 10 HOURS

Your own homemade chicken stock tastes nothing like the canned or boxed stocks you can buy in the store. The flavor is richer, the color is prettier, and you know it is completely pure and made with whole ingredients. Freeze this stock in 2-cup portions and use it in soups, stews, and sauces.

6 bone-in, skinless
   chicken thighs

2 celery stalks, cut into
   2-inch pieces

2 large carrots, cut into
   2-inch chunks

1 onion, cut into 6 wedges

12 cups water

1 teaspoon peppercorns

½ teaspoon salt

1 bay leaf

D Dairy-Free
G Gluten-Free
N Nut-Free

1 In a 6-quart slow cooker, mix all the ingredients. Cover the slow cooker and cook on low for 7 to 10 hours.

2 Remove the solids using tongs and discard. Strain the stock through cheesecloth into a large bowl.

3 Divide the stock into 2-cup portions and freeze up to 3 months.

COOKING TIP
A broth is made from vegetables and meats, but no bones. Stock is made from vegetables and meats that contain bones. Stock is richer than broth, with more flavor, and it will thicken as it cools.

NUTRITION INFORMATION
Calories: 40; Carbohydrates: 1g;
Sugar: 0g; Fiber: 0g; Fat: 2g;
Saturated Fat: 1g; Protein: 4g;
Sodium: 51mg

BEEF STOCK

MAKES 14 CUPS; SERVING SIZE ½ CUP // PREP TIME: 15 MINUTES
COOK TIME: 9 ½ TO 12 ½ HOURS

This beef stock is so good, with wonderfully rich flavor and deep and pure color. You can defat this stock before you freeze it. Put it in the fridge overnight. In the morning, remove the solid layer of fat that forms on top and discard.

4 pounds beef bones

3 carrots, cut into
    2-inch chunks

2 celery stalks, cut into
    2-inch pieces

2 onions, cut into
    8 wedges each

3 garlic cloves, peeled
    and smashed

1 tablespoon freshly squeezed
    lemon juice

1 teaspoon black peppercorns

1 teaspoon salt

1 bay leaf

12 cups water

D Dairy-Free

G Gluten-Free

N Nut-Free

1 For the richest flavor, brown the beef bones before you make the stock. In a large roasting pan, bake at 375°F for 30 to 40 minutes until they are browned.

2 In a 6-quart slow cooker, add the bones and remaining ingredients. Cover the slow cooker and cook on low for 9 to 12 hours, or until the stock is a rich brown color.

3 Remove the solids using tongs and discard. Strain the stock through cheesecloth into a large bowl.

4 Divide the stock into 2-cup portions and freeze up to 3 months.

INGREDIENT TIP
The best bones to use for this stock are oxtails, soup bones, and knucklebones. Ask the butcher for recommendations. He may even give you some bones for free!

NUTRITION INFORMATION
Calories 80; Carbohydrates: 2g;
Sugar: 1g; Fiber: 0g; Fat 5g;
Saturated Fat: 2g; Protein 7g;
Sodium: 183mg

FISH STOCK

MAKES 12 CUPS; SERVING SIZE ½ CUP // PREP TIME: 15 MINUTES
COOK TIME: 4 TO 6 HOURS

Fish stock is a great recipe to use when making seafood dishes, because it is delicate and light and really enhances the flavor of the recipe. Ask a fishmonger for shrimp shells, crab shells, and fish bones to make this excellent recipe.

2 pounds shrimp shells, fish bones, and crab shells

½ cup chopped leek

11 cups water

1 tablespoon freshly squeezed lemon juice

1 onion, cut into 4 wedges

5 garlic cloves, peeled and smashed

½ teaspoon white peppercorns

½ teaspoon salt

1 (14-ounce) BPA-free can diced tomatoes, undrained

½ teaspoon dried thyme leaves

1 In a 6-quart slow cooker, mix all the ingredients. Cover and cook on low for 4 to 6 hours. Do not cook this stock recipe longer, or it may become bitter.

2 Remove the solids using tongs and discard. Strain the stock through cheesecloth into a large bowl.

3 Divide the stock into 1-cup portions and freeze up to 3 months.

INGREDIENT TIP
Is there someone in your family who loves to fish? Have them save fish heads to make this recipe. Freeze them until you have enough to make the stock. Only use fish such as halibut or perch that are non-oily with white flesh.

Ⓓ Dairy-Free

Ⓖ Gluten-Free

Ⓝ Nut-Free

NUTRITION INFORMATION
Calories: 63; Carbohydrates: 2g; Sugar: 1g; Fiber: 0g; Fat: 2g; Saturated Fat: 2g; Protein: 8g; Sodium: 234mg

BONE BROTH

MAKES 16 CUPS; SERVING SIZE 1 CUP // PREP TIME: 15 MINUTES
COOK TIME: 8 ½ TO 10 ½ HOURS

Bone broth is technically a stock, but it's called "broth" because of alliteration, I suppose. This broth is very nutritious and is a staple of the Paleo diet because it contains large amounts of certain amino acids and glycosaminoglycans—carbohydrates that may reduce the pain of arthritis. It is a very rich base for soups and stews.

4 pounds beef bones

4 carrots, chopped

3 celery stalks, chopped

2 onions, chopped

6 garlic cloves, smashed

1 teaspoon black peppercorns

1 bay leaf

2 tablespoons freshly
    squeezed lemon juice

1 teaspoon salt

14 cups water

Ⓓ Dairy-Free

Ⓖ Gluten-Free

Ⓝ Nut-Free

NUTRITION INFORMATION
Calories: 145; Carbohydrates: 3g;
Sugar: 1g; Fiber 1g; Fat: 8g;
Saturated Fat: 3g; Protein: 13g;
Sodium: 325mg

1 In a large roasting pan, roast the bones at 400°F for about 20 to 25 minutes, or until browned.

2 In a 6-quart slow cooker, add the bones and the remaining ingredients.

3 Cover and cook on low for 8 to 10 hours, or until the broth is a deep brown.

4 Remove the solids using tongs and discard. Strain the broth through cheesecloth into a very large bowl.

5 Refrigerate the broth overnight. Remove the fat that rises to the surface and discard.

6 Divide the broth into 1-cup portions and freeze up to 3 months.

COOKING TIP
To thaw this broth or any broth or stock, put it into the fridge overnight. You can also put the frozen broth into a saucepan over low heat until it starts to melt. Add it to recipes as directed.

ROASTED VEGETABLE BROTH

MAKES 12 CUPS; SERVING SIZE 1 CUP // PREP TIME: 20 MINUTES
COOK TIME: 6 HOURS 15 MINUTES TO 8 HOURS 15 MINUTES

Vegetable broth is the ideal staple to use in vegetarian soups. Because the vegetables are roasted before the broth is made, the flavor is rich and the color is deep. But you don't have to roast the vegetables before you make this recipe; you can also just add them straight to the slow cooker.

2 onions, peeled and chopped

1 leek, chopped

3 carrots, cut into
    2-inch pieces

2 celery stalks, cut into
    2-inch pieces

4 garlic cloves, smashed

1 tablespoon olive oil

1 tablespoon freshly squeezed
    lemon juice

1 bay leaf

½ teaspoon salt

10 cups water

Ⓓ Dairy-Free
Ⓖ Gluten-Free
Ⓝ Nut-Free
Ⓥ Vegan

1 In a large roasting pan, mix the onions, leek, carrots, celery, and garlic. Drizzle with the olive oil and toss to coat. Roast at 375°F for 15 to 20 minutes, or until the vegetables are light brown.

2 In a 6-quart slow cooker, add the vegetables and remaining ingredients. Cover the slow cooker and cook on low for 6 to 8 hours.

3 Remove the solids using tongs and discard. Strain the broth through cheesecloth into a large bowl.

4 Divide the broth into 1-cup portions and freeze up to 3 months.

RECIPE TIP
Don't use starchy vegetables such as squash or potatoes when you make broth, because they will make the broth cloudy. Other vegetables such as broccoli, kale, collard greens, and cabbage add a bitter flavor to broth and should not be used.

NUTRITION INFORMATION
Calories: 30; Carbohydrates: 5g;
Sugar: 2g; Fiber: 1g; Fat: 1g;
Saturated Fat: 0g; Protein: 1g;
Sodium: 117mg

MARINARA SAUCE

MAKES 12 CUPS; SERVING SIZE 1 CUP // PREP TIME: 20 MINUTES
COOK TIME: 6 TO 8 HOURS

Marinara sauce is a classic Italian sauce usually served over spaghetti. It is made using just vegetables and herbs, and it freezes beautifully. Marinara sauce is wonderful to have on hand in the freezer; just heat it up and serve over hot cooked pasta for a quick dinner.

4 pounds Roma tomatoes, chopped

4 beefsteak tomatoes, seeded and chopped

1 (6-ounce) can BPA-free tomato paste

2 onions, peeled and chopped

4 garlic cloves, peeled and minced

½ cup shredded carrot

1 bay leaf

2 teaspoons dried basil leaves

1 teaspoon dried oregano leaves

1 In a 6-quart slow cooker, mix all the ingredients. Cover and cook on low for 6 to 8 hours.

2 Remove and discard the bay leaf.

3 You can freeze this sauce as is, or you can puree it by using a potato masher to crush some of the tomatoes.

4 Divide the sauce into 2-cup portions and freeze up to 4 months.

INGREDIENT TIP
Canned tomato paste is essential to making this sauce rich and flavorful. Make sure that the tomato paste you purchase is in BPA-free cans. You can usually find that product at co-ops and health food stores.

D Dairy-Free
G Gluten-Free
N Nut-Free
V Vegan

NUTRITION INFORMATION
Calories: 77; Carbohydrates: 16g;
Sugar: 8g; Fiber: 4g; Fat: 1g;
Saturated Fat: 0g; Protein: 3g;
Sodium: 19mg

BOLOGNESE SAUCE

MAKES 12 CUPS; SERVING SIZE 1 CUP // PREP TIME: 20 MINUTES
COOK TIME: 7 TO 9 HOURS

Bolognese sauce is a rich Italian sauce made with ground beef. It is usually made with red wine and milk. We'll omit the wine, and use diced mushrooms for a rich flavor. Serve this sauce over pasta or use it to make the best lasagna ever.

2 pounds lean grass-fed ground beef

2 onions, chopped

7 garlic cloves, minced

1 large carrot, grated

¼ cup tomato paste (see tip on page 31)

3 pounds Roma tomatoes, seeded and chopped

2 cups bottled tomato juice

1 bay leaf

1 teaspoon dried oregano leaves

½ teaspoon salt

D Dairy-Free
G Gluten-Free
N Nut-Free

NUTRITION INFORMATION
Calories: 167; Carbohydrates: 12g;
Sugar: 6g; Fiber: 2g; Fat: 6g;
Saturated Fat: 2g; Protein: 18g;
Sodium: 265mg

1 In a large skillet, mix the ground beef, onions, and garlic. Cook over medium heat, stirring frequently to break up the meat, until the beef is browned. Drain.

2 In a 6-quart slow cooker, mix the beef mixture with the remaining ingredients. Cover and cook on low for 7 to 9 hours, or until the sauce is thickened.

3 Remove the bay leaf and discard.

4 Divide the sauce into 3-cup portions and freeze up to 3 months. To use, let the sauce thaw in the refrigerator overnight, then slowly heat in a saucepan until the sauce is bubbling.

INGREDIENT TIP
Grass-fed beef is better for you than beef that is raised on corn. Grass-fed beef has a good ratio of omega-3 to omega-6 fats and it's also a good source of a type of fat that may reduce the risk of cancer. Omega-6 fatty acids are pro-inflammatory, which means they can irritate the cells in your body.

ROASTED TOMATO SAUCE

MAKES 13 CUPS SAUCE; SERVING SIZE 1 CUP // PREP TIME: 20 MINUTES
COOK TIME: 9 TO 11 HOURS

Roasting tomatoes right in the slow cooker is an easy step that really adds to the richness and flavor of this sauce. You don't add anything to the tomatoes in the first step: no olive oil, no salt, no herbs. This step helps concentrate the tomatoes. Then you add the remaining ingredients and cook until the sauce is thick and rich.

4 pounds Roma tomatoes, seeded and chopped

2 onions, chopped

5 garlic cloves, minced

3 tablespoons extra-virgin olive oil

2 cups bottled tomato juice

3 tablespoons tomato paste (see tip below and on page 31)

2 teaspoons dried basil leaves

½ teaspoon salt

⅛ teaspoon white pepper

D Dairy-Free

G Gluten-Free

N Nut-Free

V Vegan

NUTRITION INFORMATION
Calories: 76; Carbohydrates: 11g; Sugar: 6g; Fiber: 2g; Fat: 3g; Saturated Fat: 0g; Protein: 2g; Sodium: 210mg

1 In a 6-quart slow cooker, place all the tomatoes. Partially cover the slow cooker and cook the tomatoes on high for 3 hours, stirring the tomatoes twice during cooking time.

2 Add the remaining ingredients. Cover and cook on low for 6 to 8 hours longer, until the sauce is bubbling and the consistency you want.

3 You can make the sauce smoother if you'd like by working the sauce with a potato masher, or leave it as is.

4 Divide the sauce into 2-cup portions and freeze up to 3 months.

INGREDIENT TIP
You can sometimes find tomato paste in squeeze bottles. That is a great way to be able to use a few tablespoons of tomato paste without having to open a can. Just store the opened bottle in the refrigerator.

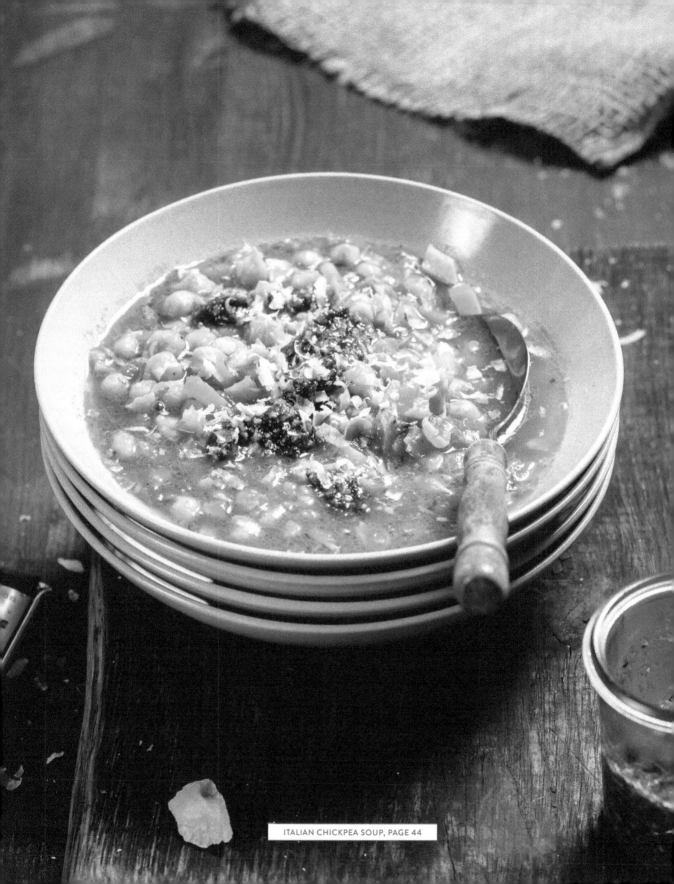

ITALIAN CHICKPEA SOUP, PAGE 44

CHAPTER THREE

BEANS AND GRAINS

BARLEY RISOTTO

SERVES 8 // PREP TIME: 15 MINUTES // COOK TIME: 7 TO 8 HOURS

Risotto is typically made with rice. The grain is slowly cooked with wine and broth until the rice releases starch and the mixture becomes creamy. This version is made with barley, which means you don't have to stir as the mixture cooks, and barley is healthier than rice. Enjoy this recipe with a green salad and some fresh fruit.

2¼ cups hulled barley, rinsed

1 onion, finely chopped

4 garlic cloves, minced

1 (8-ounce) package button mushrooms, chopped

6 cups low-sodium vegetable broth

½ teaspoon dried marjoram leaves

⅛ teaspoon freshly ground black pepper

⅔ cup grated Parmesan cheese

1 In a 6-quart slow cooker, mix the barley, onion, garlic, mushrooms, broth, marjoram, and pepper. Cover and cook on low for 7 to 8 hours, or until the barley has absorbed most of the liquid and is tender, and the vegetables are tender.

2 Stir in the Parmesan cheese and serve.

INGREDIENT TIP
There are several types of barley available in the store. Hulled barley is minimally processed and contains the bran layer, so it is considered a whole grain. Pearl barley has had the bran layer removed. It is not considered a whole grain. Hulled barley takes longer to cook than pearl barley.

N Nut-Free

V Vegetarian

NUTRITION INFORMATION
Calories: 288; Carbohydrates: 45g; Sugar: 2g; Fiber: 9g; Fat: 6g; Saturated Fat: 3g; Protein: 13g; Sodium: 495mg

RISOTTO WITH GREEN BEANS, SWEET POTATOES, AND PEAS

SERVES 8 // PREP TIME: 20 MINUTES // COOK TIME: 4 TO 5 HOURS

Risotto is such an elegant dish that is so easy to cook in the slow cooker. It can be a side dish, or it can be the meal. With the addition of sweet potatoes, beans, and peas, this dish would be perfect for a light lunch or a vegetarian main dish.

1 large sweet potato, peeled and chopped

1 onion, chopped

5 garlic cloves, minced

2 cups short-grain brown rice

1 teaspoon dried thyme leaves

7 cups low-sodium vegetable broth

2 cups green beans, cut in half crosswise

2 cups frozen baby peas

3 tablespoons unsalted butter

½ cup grated Parmesan cheese

1 In a 6-quart slow cooker, mix the sweet potato, onion, garlic, rice, thyme, and broth. Cover and cook on low for 3 to 4 hours, or until the rice is tender.

2 Stir in the green beans and frozen peas. Cover and cook on low for 30 to 40 minutes or until the vegetables are tender.

3 Stir in the butter and cheese. Cover and cook on low for 20 minutes, then stir and serve.

INGREDIENT TIP
Baby peas are much more tender and sweeter than regular frozen peas. You can use regular peas if you'd like. This vegetable thaws and cooks very quickly in the slow cooker, so the peas will be tender and hot at the same time it takes the beans to cook.

G Gluten-Free

N Nut-Free

V Vegetarian

NUTRITION INFORMATION
Calories: 385; Carbohydrates: 52g;
Sugar: 4g; Fiber: 6g; Fat: 10g;
Saturated Fat: 5g; Protein: 10g;
Sodium: 426mg

THREE-BEAN MEDLEY

SERVES 8 // PREP TIME: 15 MINUTES // COOK TIME: 6 TO 8 HOURS

Dried beans and the slow cooker are made for each other. And dried beans are about as clean an ingredient as you can find! This pantry staple is full of fiber.

1¼ cups dried kidney beans, rinsed and drained

1¼ cups dried black beans, rinsed and drained

1¼ cups dried black-eyed peas, rinsed and drained

1 onion, chopped

1 leek, chopped

2 garlic cloves, minced

2 carrots, peeled and chopped

6 cups low-sodium vegetable broth

1½ cups water

½ teaspoon dried thyme leaves

In a 6-quart slow cooker, mix all of the ingredients. Cover and cook on low for 6 to 8 hours, or until the beans are tender and the liquid is absorbed.

INGREDIENT TIP
Many recipes call for soaking dried beans before cooking them; but that's just not necessary. Soaking does not reduce the gassiness some people get from beans. And unsoaked beans have a better texture and more flavor. So just rinse the dried beans and cook them.

D Dairy-Free
G Gluten-Free
N Nut-Free
V Vegan

NUTRITION INFORMATION
Calories: 284; Carbohydrates: 56g;
Sugar: 6g; Fiber: 19g; Fat: 0g;
Saturated Fat: 0g; Protein: 19g;
Sodium: 131mg

HERBED GARLIC BLACK BEANS

SERVES 8 // PREP TIME: 10 MINUTES // COOK TIME: 7 TO 9 HOURS

Black beans, also called turtle beans, have a black coating, but their interior is creamy and white. They are velvety with a meaty flavor when cooked, so they are a great meat substitute for vegetarians and vegans. Cooked with herbs and garlic, they are a flavorful treat.

3 cups dried black beans, rinsed and drained

2 onions, chopped

8 garlic cloves, minced

6 cups low-sodium vegetable broth

½ teaspoon salt

1 teaspoon dried basil leaves

½ teaspoon dried thyme leaves

½ teaspoon dried oregano leaves

1 In a 6-quart slow cooker, mix all the ingredients. Cover and cook on low for 7 to 9 hours, or until the beans have absorbed the liquid and are tender.

2 Remove and discard the bay leaf.

VARIATION TIP
You can make this recipe with any type of dried bean. Pinto beans, which are a creamy color with mottled red spots, are delicious when cooked this way. Cannellini or great northern beans are also a good substitute.

D Dairy-Free
G Gluten-Free
N Nut-Free
V Vegan

NUTRITION INFORMATION
Calories: 250; Carbohydrates: 47g;
Sugar: 3g; Fiber: 17g; Fat: 0g;
Saturated Fat: 0g; Protein: 15g;
Sodium: 253mg

QUINOA WITH VEGETABLES

SERVES 8 // PREP TIME: 10 MINUTES // COOK TIME: 5 TO 6 HOURS

Quinoa (pronounced "keen-wah") is an ancient whole grain (actually a seed) that is gluten-free and high in protein. It contains all of the amino acids necessary to live. It's also high in B vitamins, calcium, magnesium, and vitamin E. It's delicious when cooked with vegetables and has a nutty flavor and chewy texture.

2 cups quinoa, rinsed and drained

2 onions, chopped

2 carrots, peeled and sliced

1 cup sliced cremini mushrooms

3 garlic cloves, minced

4 cups low-sodium vegetable broth

½ teaspoon salt

1 teaspoon dried marjoram leaves

⅛ teaspoon freshly ground black pepper

1 In a 6-quart slow cooker, mix all of the ingredients. Cover and cook on low for 5 to 6 hours, or until the quinoa and vegetables are tender.

2 Stir the mixture and serve.

INGREDIENT TIP
Quinoa has a sticky, bitter coating made of a compound called saponin. This chemical helps protect the seed from insects while it's growing. Rinse quinoa well before you cook it to get rid of the saponin.

D Dairy-Free
G Gluten-Free
N Nut-Free
V Vegan

NUTRITION INFORMATION
Calories: 204; Carbohydrates: 35g;
Sugar: 4g; Fiber: 4g; Fat: 3g;
Saturated Fat: 0g; Protein: 7g;
Sodium: 229mg

HERBED WILD RICE

SERVES 8 // PREP TIME: 10 MINUTES // COOK TIME: 4 TO 6 HOURS

Wild rice is perfect for the slow cooker. This grass seed is grown in shallow marshes in the northern part of Minnesota. It is traditionally harvested by men in canoes who glide through the marshes, gently bending the stalks of the grass and removing the seeds. It is delicious, with a nutty taste and slightly chewy texture.

3 cups wild rice, rinsed and drained

6 cups Roasted Vegetable Broth (page 30)

1 onion, chopped

½ teaspoon salt

½ teaspoon dried thyme leaves

½ teaspoon dried basil leaves

1 bay leaf

⅓ cup chopped fresh flat-leaf parsley

1 In a 6-quart slow cooker, mix the wild rice, vegetable broth, onion, salt, thyme, basil, and bay leaf. Cover and cook on low for 4 to 6 hours, or until the wild rice is tender but still firm. You can cook this dish longer until the wild rice pops; that will take about 7 to 8 hours.

2 Remove and discard the bay leaf.

3 Stir in the parsley and serve.

INGREDIENT TIP
When you buy wild rice in the store, look for naturally harvested wild rice to support local Indian tribes, and make sure that the grains are long and whole. Broken grains will cook up mushy.

D Dairy-Free
G Gluten-Free
N Nut-Free
V Vegan

NUTRITION INFORMATION
Calories: 258; Carbohydrates: 54g; Sugar: 3g; Fiber: 5g; Fat: 2g; Saturated Fat: 0g; Protein: 6g; Sodium: 257mg

GARLIC LENTILS

SERVES 8 // PREP TIME: 10 MINUTES // COOK TIME: 4 TO 5 HOURS

Most lentils are perfect for the slow cooker. There are several types of lentils on the market. Green lentils are a mottled brown with green and have a slightly spicy flavor. Puy lentils, which are considered the best in flavor and texture, are green. These take the longest to cook. Brown lentils are the most common and have a mild flavor. And red lentils are nutty and sweet but not the best choice for the slow cooker.

3 cups puy lentils, rinsed and drained

1 onion, chopped

1 leek, chopped

8 garlic cloves, minced

6 cups Roasted Vegetable Broth (page 30)

1 bay leaf

½ teaspoon dried oregano leaves

1 In a 6-quart slow cooker, mix all the ingredients. Cover and cook on low for 4 to 5 hours, or until the lentils are tender.

2 Remove and discard the bay leaf.

VARIATION TIP
Stir these cooked lentils into any soup or stew you are making, or puree them in a food processor with some lemon juice, herbs, and olive oil for a healthy appetizer dip.

D Dairy-Free
G Gluten-Free
N Nut-Free
V Vegan

NUTRITION INFORMATION
Calories: 208; Carbohydrates: 36g;
Sugar: 5g; Fiber: 17g; Fat: 0g;
Saturated Fat: 0g; Protein: 16g;
Sodium: 109mg

BARLEY AND BLACK BEANS

SERVES 10 // PREP TIME: 15 MINUTES // COOK TIME: 7 TO 8 HOURS

Barley and black beans is a classic vegetarian combination that makes a great side dish. The mixture of tender barley and slightly sweet black beans is delicious. You must use hulled barley in this recipe; the pearl variety cooks too quickly and will be mushy by the time the beans are done.

2 cups dried black beans, rinsed and drained

1½ cups hulled barley

1 onion, chopped

3 garlic cloves, minced

8 cups Roasted Vegetable Broth (page 30)

1 bay leaf

½ teaspoon dried thyme leaves

D Dairy-Free
N Nut-Free
V Vegan

NUTRITION INFORMATION
Calories: 240; Carbohydrates: 46g;
Sugar: 2g; Fiber: 14g; Fat: 1g;
Saturated Fat: 0g; Protein: 12g;
Sodium: 115mg

1 In a 6-quart slow cooker, mix all of the ingredients. Cover and cook on low for 7 to 8 hours, or until the barley and black beans are tender.

2 Remove and discard the bay leaf.

VARIATION TIP
You can use this mixture to make a quick soup. Just mix about 2 cups of it with more vegetable broth and add some sliced carrots and some chopped bell peppers. Simmer for about 5 to 10 minutes, then eat!

ITALIAN CHICKPEA SOUP

SERVES 8 // PREP TIME: 20 MINUTES // COOK TIME: 5 TO 6 HOURS

This classic soup is so heartwarming and comforting. The flavors are delicious, and the texture of the chickpeas is perfect against the soft carrots and onions. Parsley root is a root vegetable that looks like a wrinkled white carrot and has a wonderful flavor of, well, parsley! If you can't find it, substitute one turnip or rutabaga.

2 onions, chopped

3 garlic cloves, minced

4 carrots, peeled and cut into chunks

2 medium parsley roots, peeled and sliced

2 (14-ounce) BPA-free cans diced tomatoes, undrained

2 (15-ounce) BPA-free cans no-salt-added chickpeas, drained and rinsed

6 cups Roasted Vegetable Broth (page 30)

1 teaspoon dried basil leaves

¼ teaspoon freshly ground black pepper

1 In a 6-quart slow cooker, layer all of the ingredients. Cover and cook on low for 5 to 6 hours, or until the vegetables are tender.

2 Stir the soup and serve topped with pesto, if desired.

INGREDIENT TIP

To make pesto, mix 2 cups fresh basil leaves and 1 garlic clove in a blender or food processor; blend or process until finely chopped. With the motor running, add ⅓ cup extra-virgin olive oil until well combined. Stir in ⅓ cup grated Parmesan cheese and season with salt and pepper.

D Dairy-Free

G Gluten-Free

N Nut-Free

V Vegan

NUTRITION INFORMATION

Calorie: 154; Carbohydrates: 30g; Sugar: 10g; Fiber: 6g; Fat: 2g; Saturated Fat: 0g; Protein: 6g; Sodium: 469mg

ROSEMARY WHITE BEANS

SERVES 16 // PREP TIME: 15 MINUTES // COOK TIME: 6 TO 8 HOURS

White beans cook beautifully in the slow cooker. You can use them in many ways—as a side dish, as an addition to a quick soup, or mash them for an appetizer dip. These beans are flavored with fresh rosemary leaves, onion, and garlic.

1 pound great northern beans

1 onion, finely chopped

3 cloves garlic, minced

1 large sprig fresh rosemary

½ teaspoon salt

⅛ teaspoon white pepper

4 cups water

2 cups low sodium
   vegetable broth

D Dairy-Free
G Gluten-Free
N Nut-Free
V Vegan

1 Sort over the beans and remove any extraneous material. Rinse the beans well and drain.

2 Combine the beans, onion, garlic, rosemary, salt, water, and vegetable broth in a 6-quart slow cooker.

3 Cover and cook on low for 6 to 8 hours or until the beans are tender.

4 Remove the rosemary stem and discard. Stir the mixture gently and serve.

SUBSTITUTION TIP:
You can use other dried white beans in place of the great northern beans in this easy recipe. Dried cannellini beans (also known as white kidney beans) and navy beans will work well in this recipe.

NUTRITION INFORMATION
Calories: 88; Carbohydrates: 17g;
Sugar: 0g; Fiber: 5g; Fat: 0g;
Saturated Fat: 0g; Protein: 5g;
Sodium: 362mg

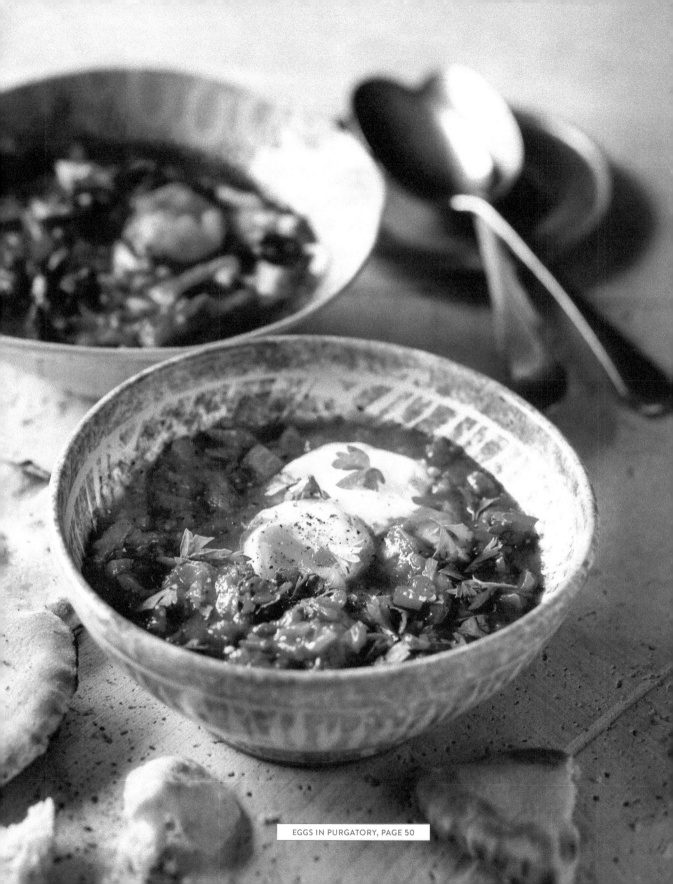

EGGS IN PURGATORY, PAGE 50

CHAPTER FOUR

BREAKFAST AND BRUNCH

SAVORY BASIL OATMEAL

SERVES 8 // PREP TIME: 10 MINUTES // COOK TIME: 7 TO 8 HOURS

Savory oatmeal is a nice change of pace from sweet oatmeal in the mornings, and it's much better for you. All the sugar that is usually added to slow cooker oatmeal doesn't provide any nutrition, and it increases the calories.

3 cups steel-cut oatmeal

2 shallots, peeled and minced

5 cups Roasted Vegetable Broth (page 30)

1 cup water

1 teaspoon dried basil leaves

½ teaspoon dried thyme leaves

¼ teaspoon salt

¼ teaspoon freshly ground black pepper

½ cup grated Parmesan cheese

2 cups chopped baby spinach leaves

2 tablespoons chopped fresh basil

1 In a 6-quart slow cooker, mix the oatmeal, shallots, vegetable broth, water, basil, thyme, salt, and pepper. Cover and cook on low for 7 to 8 hours, or until the oatmeal is tender.

2 Stir in the Parmesan cheese, spinach, and basil, and let stand, covered, for another 5 minutes. Stir and serve.

INGREDIENT TIP
Steel-cut oatmeal is different from quick cooking and regular oatmeal. The whole oat is simply cut into pieces, so it cooks much more slowly and still has a slightly chewy texture after hours in the slow cooker.

(G) Gluten-Free

(N) Nut-Free

(V) Vegetarian

NUTRITION INFORMATION
Calories: 262; Carbohydrates: 43g;
Sugar: 2g; Fiber: 6g; Fat: 5g;
Saturated Fat: 2g; Protein: 8g;
Sodium: 172mg

ROOT VEGETABLE HASH

SERVES 8 // PREP TIME: 20 MINUTES // COOK TIME: 7 TO 8 HOURS

Hash is ideal for breakfast. This combination of root vegetables is tender and slightly sweet. Top it with a poached or fried egg if you'd like, but you can eat this hash all on its own. Serve with a slice of toasted low-sodium whole-wheat bread (see tip on page 57) and enjoy.

4 Yukon Gold
   potatoes, chopped

2 russet potatoes, chopped

1 large parsnip, peeled
   and chopped

3 large carrots, peeled
   and chopped

2 onions, chopped

2 garlic cloves, minced

2 tablespoons olive oil

¼ cup Roasted Vegetable
   Broth (page 30)

½ teaspoon salt

1 teaspoon dried thyme leaves

1 In a 6-quart slow cooker, mix all of the ingredients. Cover and cook on low for 7 to 8 hours.

2 Stir the hash well and serve.

VARIATION TIP
Any leftovers of this hash can be made into crisp vegetable cakes. Just mix 2 cups of the hash with 3 tablespoons whole-wheat flour and 1 egg. Make into small cakes, then fry in some olive oil, turning once, until they're crisp.

Ⓓ Dairy-Free
Ⓖ Gluten-Free
Ⓝ Nut-Free
Ⓥ Vegan

NUTRITION INFORMATION
Calories: 150; Carbohydrates: 28g;
Sugar: 4g; Fiber: 4g; Fat: 4g;
Saturated Fat: 0g; Protein: 3g;
Sodium: 176mg

EGGS IN PURGATORY

SERVES 8 // PREP TIME: 15 MINUTES // COOK TIME: 7 TO 8 HOURS

Eggs in Purgatory are simply eggs that are poached in a slightly spicy tomato sauce. The sauce cooks all night in your slow cooker, then the eggs are added during the last 20 minutes of cooking. This is an unusual breakfast recipe that will wake up your taste buds!

2½ pounds Roma
   tomatoes, chopped

2 onions, chopped

2 garlic cloves, chopped

1 teaspoon paprika

½ teaspoon ground cumin

½ teaspoon dried
   marjoram leaves

1 cup Roasted Vegetable
   Broth (page 30)

8 large eggs

2 red chili peppers, minced

½ cup chopped
   flat-leaf parsley

G Gluten-Free

N Nut-Free

V Vegetarian

NUTRITION INFORMATION
Calories: 116; Carbohydrates: 10g;
Sugar: 5g; Fiber: 2g; Fat: 5g;
Saturated Fat: 2g; Protein: 8g;
Sodium: 102mg

1 In a 6-quart slow cooker, mix the tomatoes, onions, garlic, paprika, cumin, marjoram, and vegetable broth, and stir to mix. Cover and cook on low for 7 to 8 hours, or until a sauce has formed.

2 One at a time, break the eggs into the sauce; do not stir.

3 Cover and cook on high until the egg whites are completely set and the yolk is thickened, about 20 minutes. Sprinkle the eggs with the minced red chili peppers.

4 Sprinkle with the parsley and serve.

INGREDIENT TIP
If anyone in your family is in a high-risk group for food poisoning, consider using pasteurized eggs. Eggs should always be cooked well done. In this recipe, the eggs are not quite cooked to 160°F. You can cook the eggs until the yolks are firm.

THREE-GRAIN GRANOLA

MAKES 20 CUPS; SERVES 40 // PREP TIME: 15 MINUTES // COOK TIME: 3½ TO 5 HOURS

Your own homemade granola is going to be so much better, in terms of flavor, nutrition, and saving money, than anything you can buy at the store. You can use any type of flaked grain you'd like in this easy recipe and vary the dried fruits too. By the way, buckwheat does not contain gluten, despite the "wheat" in its name. Buckwheat is related to rhubarb.

5 cups regular oatmeal

4 cups barley flakes

3 cups buckwheat flakes

2 cups whole almonds

2 cups whole walnuts

½ cup honey

2 teaspoons ground cinnamon

1 tablespoon vanilla extract

2 cups golden raisins

2 cups dried cherries

Ⓓ Dairy-Free
Ⓥ Vegetarian

NUTRITION INFORMATION
Calories: 214; Carbohydrates: 33g; Sugar: 13g; Fiber: 4g; Fat: 8g; Saturated Fat: 1g; Protein: 6g; Sodium: 17mg

1 In a 6-quart slow cooker, mix the oatmeal, barley flakes, buckwheat flakes, almonds, and walnuts.

2 In a small bowl, mix the honey, cinnamon, and vanilla, and mix well. Drizzle this mixture over the food in the slow cooker and stir with a spatula to coat.

3 Partially cover the slow cooker. Cook on low for 3½ to 5 hours, stirring twice during cooking time, until the oatmeal, barley and buckwheat flakes, and nuts are toasted.

4 Remove the granola from the slow cooker and spread on two large baking sheets. Add the raisins and cherries to the granola and stir gently.

5 Let the granola cool, then store in an airtight container at room temperature.

INGREDIENT TIP
Barley flakes are made just like oatmeal, but are made from barley instead. Their flavor is sweet and nutty, and when cooked in liquid, they remain slightly chewy. And buckwheat flakes are made the same way.

BAKED BERRY OATMEAL

SERVES 12 // PREP TIME: 15 MINUTES // COOK TIME: 4 TO 6 HOURS

Baked oatmeal contains eggs and milk, so it will set into a mixture that can be cut into squares. This recipe resembles an oatmeal cookie, but it's much better for you. Serve it with some maple syrup or honey drizzled over each piece.

7 cups rolled oats

4 eggs

1½ cups almond milk

2 tablespoons melted coconut oil

⅓ cup honey

¼ teaspoon salt

1 teaspoon ground cinnamon

¼ teaspoon ground ginger

1½ cups dried blueberries

1 cup dried cherries

D Dairy-Free
G Gluten-Free
V Vegetarian

NUTRITION INFORMATION
Calories: 368; Carbohydrates: 68g;
Sugar: 33g; Fiber: 6g; Fat: 7g;
Saturated Fat: 3g; Protein: 9g;
Sodium: 97mg

1 Grease a 6-quart slow cooker with plain vegetable oil.

2 In a large bowl, place the rolled oats.

3 In a medium bowl, mix the eggs, almond milk, coconut oil, honey, salt, cinnamon, and ginger. Mix until well combined. Pour this mixture over the oats.

4 Gently stir in the dried blueberries and dried cherries. Pour into the prepared slow cooker.

5 Cover and cook on low for 4 to 6 hours, or until the oatmeal mixture is set and the edges start to brown.

VARIATION TIP
Leftovers of this recipe can be crumbled on top of yogurt for breakfast. Try it with plain Greek yogurt and add some sliced strawberries or blueberries for a great start to the day.

CRANBERRY-QUINOA HOT CEREAL

SERVES 12 // PREP TIME: 15 MINUTES // COOK TIME: 6 TO 8 HOURS

Quinoa, the whole grain that is a complete protein, makes a fabulous breakfast cereal. It becomes creamy and stays slightly chewy when cooked in the slow cooker. Dried cranberries add a burst of color and pop of flavor to this excellent recipe.

3 cups quinoa, rinsed and drained

2 cups unsweetened apple juice

4 cups canned coconut milk

2 cups water

¼ cup honey

1 teaspoon vanilla extract

1 teaspoon ground cinnamon

½ teaspoon salt

1½ cups dried cranberries (see tip on page 68)

In a 6-quart slow cooker, mix all of the ingredients. Cover and cook on low for 6 to 8 hours or until the quinoa is creamy.

VARIATION TIP
You can use just about any liquid you'd like when you cook cereal in the slow cooker. Use unsweetened pineapple juice, soy milk, almond milk, or plain old cow's milk. It just depends on what you like to eat and your taste.

Ⓓ Dairy-Free
Ⓖ Gluten-Free
Ⓥ Vegetarian

NUTRITION INFORMATION
Calories: 284; Carbohydrates: 55g;
Sugar: 25g; Fiber: 4g; Fat: 4g;
Saturated Fat: 1g; Protein: 6g;
Sodium: 104mg

MEDITERRANEAN STRATA

SERVES 10 // PREP TIME: 20 MINUTES // COOK TIME: 5 TO 7 HOURS

The foods of the Mediterranean include olive oil, garlic, lemons, olives, oregano, mint, red peppers, and nuts. Some of these ingredients are mixed with bread, eggs, and milk to make this savory breakfast strata. The Mediterranean diet, by the way, is considered one of the healthiest in the world.

8 cups whole-wheat bread (see tip on page 57), cut into cubes

1 onion, finely chopped

3 garlic cloves, minced

2 red bell peppers, stemmed, seeded, and chopped

2 cups chopped baby spinach leaves

4 eggs

2 egg whites

2 tablespoons olive oil

1½ cups 2% milk

1 cup shredded Asiago cheese

1 In a 6-quart slow cooker, mix the bread cubes, onion, garlic, bell peppers, and spinach.

2 In a medium bowl, mix the eggs, egg whites, olive oil, and milk, and beat well. Pour this mixture into the slow cooker. Sprinkle with the cheese.

3 Cover and cook on low for 5 to 7 hours, or until a food thermometer registers 165°F and the strata is set and puffed.

4 Scoop the strata out of the slow cooker to serve.

SUBSTITUTION TIP
You can substitute a can of artichoke hearts for the red bell peppers if you'd like. Just drain them and cut each heart into four to six pieces. You can also use kale or other dark leafy green in place of the spinach in this recipe.

N Nut-Free

V Vegetarian

NUTRITION INFORMATION
Calories: 385; Carbohydrates: 55g;
Sugar: 11g; Fiber: 8g; Fat: 11g;
Saturated Fat: 3g; Protein: 16g;
Sodium: 672mg

MIXED BERRY HONEY GRANOLA

MAKES 20 CUPS; SERVING SIZE ½ CUP // PREP TIME: 15 MINUTES
COOK TIME: 3½ TO 5 HOURS

You can serve granola as is, use it as a topping for yogurt or to add some crunch to hot cereal, eat it as a snack, or cook it to make another type of hot cereal. This recipe is very versatile. You can omit the berries, add other nuts, or add your own favorite spices.

10 cups rolled oats

2 cups whole almonds

2 cups whole walnuts

2 cups macadamia nuts

½ cup honey

2 teaspoons ground cinnamon

¼ teaspoon ground cardamom

1 tablespoon vanilla extract

2 cups dried blueberries

2 cups dried cherries

D Dairy-Free
G Gluten-Free
V Vegetarian

NUTRITION INFORMATION
Calories: 255; Carbohydrates: 33g; Sugar: 16g; Fiber: 4g; Fat: 12g; Saturated Fat: 2g; Protein: 6g; Sodium: 14mg

1 In a 6-quart slow cooker, mix the oatmeal, almonds, walnuts, and macadamia nuts.

2 In a small bowl, mix the honey, cinnamon, cardamom, and vanilla. Drizzle this mixture over the oatmeal mixture in the slow cooker and stir with a spatula to coat.

3 Partially cover the slow cooker. Cook on low for 3½ to 5 hours, stirring twice during cooking time, until the oatmeal and nuts are toasted.

4 Remove the granola from the slow cooker and spread on two large baking sheets. Add the dried blueberries and cherries to the granola and stir gently.

5 Let the granola cool, then store in an airtight container at room temperature up to one week.

INGREDIENT TIP '
Do not use quick cooking or instant oatmeal in this granola recipe, or any granola recipe for that matter. Those ingredients are not sturdy enough to stand up to the long cooking time, and the granola will be mushy.

EGG AND POTATO STRATA

SERVES 8 // PREP TIME: 20 MINUTES // COOK TIME: 6 TO 8 HOURS

A strata is usually made of bread that is soaked in an egg-and-milk mixture, then baked so it puffs and turns golden brown. Potatoes are used instead of bread in this recipe to make it gluten-free. Serve it with orange juice, coffee, and fresh fruit.

8 Yukon Gold potatoes, peeled and diced

1 onion, minced

2 red bell peppers, stemmed, seeded, and minced

3 Roma tomatoes, seeded and chopped

3 garlic cloves, minced

1½ cups shredded Swiss cheese

8 eggs

2 egg whites

1 teaspoon dried marjoram leaves

1 cup 2% milk

1 In a 6-quart slow cooker, layer the diced potatoes, onion, bell peppers, tomatoes, garlic, and cheese.

2 In a medium bowl, mix the eggs, egg whites, marjoram, and milk well with a wire whisk. Pour this mixture into the slow cooker.

3 Cover and cook on low for 6 to 8 hours, or until a food thermometer registers 165°F and the potatoes are tender.

4 Scoop out of the slow cooker to serve.

SUBSTITUTION TIP
You can substitute other types of potatoes for the Yukon Gold potatoes in this recipe. Use 6 peeled and diced russet potatoes, or mix russet potatoes and sweet potatoes.

G Gluten-Free

N Nut-Free

V Vegetarian

NUTRITION INFORMATION
Calories: 305; Carbohydrates: 33g;
Sugar: 5g; Fiber: 3g; Fat: 12g;
Saturated Fat: 6g; Protein: 17g;
Sodium: 136mg

APPLE FRENCH TOAST BAKE

SERVES 8 // PREP TIME: 20 MINUTES // COOK TIME: 4 TO 5 HOURS

This recipe has the flavors of apple pie, but in French toast form. The apples soften in the slow cooker, most of the bread gets custardy, and the edges of the bread get slightly crisp, so you get the best of both worlds. Serve this with some maple syrup for those who like their French toast a little sweeter.

¼ cup coconut sugar

1 teaspoon ground cinnamon

¼ teaspoon ground cardamom

10 slices whole-wheat bread, cubed

2 Granny Smith apples, peeled and diced

8 eggs

1 cup canned coconut milk

1 cup unsweetened apple juice

2 teaspoons vanilla extract

1 cup granola

D Dairy-Free

V Vegetarian

NUTRITION INFORMATION
Calories: 317; Carbohydrates: 49g; Sugar: 18g; Fiber: 6g; Fat: 9g; Saturated Fat: 3g; Protein: 12g; Sodium: 326mg

1 Grease a 6-quart slow cooker with plain vegetable oil.

2 In a small bowl, mix the coconut sugar, cinnamon, and cardamom well.

3 In the slow cooker, layer the bread, apples, and coconut sugar mixture.

4 In a large bowl, mix the eggs, coconut milk, apple juice, and vanilla, and mix well. Pour this mixture slowly over the food in the slow cooker. Sprinkle the granola on top.

5 Cover and cook on low for 4 to 5 hours, or until a food thermometer registers 165°F.

6 Scoop the mixture from the slow cooker to serve.

INGREDIENT TIP
Bread can be high in sodium, so if you are watching your blood pressure, choose low-sodium bread for this and other recipes. And make sure that whole-wheat flour is the first ingredient on the bread label for the best nutrition.

QUINOA-KALE-EGG CASSEROLE

SERVES 8 // PREP TIME: 20 MINUTES // COOK TIME: 6 TO 8 HOURS

Quinoa makes a great savory breakfast casserole when it's cooked with eggs, kale, bell peppers, and a few other ingredients. Eating a savory breakfast is one way to cut down on your sugar intake. And recipes like this one are much more filling than a bowl of cereal.

3 cups 2% milk

1½ cups Roasted Vegetable Broth (page 30)

11 eggs

1½ cups quinoa, rinsed and drained

3 cups chopped kale

1 leek, chopped

1 red bell pepper, stemmed, seeded, and chopped

3 garlic cloves, minced

1½ cups shredded Havarti cheese

(G) Gluten-Free

(N) Nut-Free

(V) Vegetarian

NUTRITION INFORMATION
Calories: 483; Carbohydrates: 32g; Sugar: 8g; Fiber: 3g; Fat: 27g; Saturated Fat: 14g; Protein: 25g; Sodium: 462mg

1 Grease a 6-quart slow cooker with vegetable oil and set aside.

2 In a large bowl, mix the milk, vegetable broth, and eggs, and beat well with a wire whisk.

3 Stir in the quinoa, kale, leek, bell pepper, garlic, and cheese. Pour this mixture into the prepared slow cooker.

4 Cover and cook on low for 6 to 8 hours, or until a food thermometer registers 165°F and the mixture is set.

SUBSTITUTION TIP
You can use any chopped vegetable in place of the leek and red bell pepper in this recipe. Try using chopped zucchini or yellow summer squash. Frozen peas or some corn would also be good.

CARROT CAKE OATMEAL

SERVES 8 // PREP TIME: 20 MINUTES // COOK TIME: 6 TO 8 HOURS

This recipe really does taste like carrot cake made with oatmeal, but it's not as sweet. The steel-cut oats stay slightly chewy, and the carrot softens and adds a wonderful sweet flavor to the recipe. And the pineapple caramelizes slightly around the edges of the slow cooker, adding more flavor.

3 cups steel-cut oats

2 cups finely grated carrot

1 (8-ounce) BPA-free can unsweetened crushed pineapple in juice, undrained

2 cups almond milk

4 cups water

2 tablespoons melted coconut oil

¼ cup honey

2 teaspoons vanilla extract

¼ teaspoon salt

1 teaspoon ground cinnamon

Ⓓ Dairy-Free

Ⓖ Gluten-Free

Ⓥ Vegetarian

NUTRITION INFORMATION
Calories: 132; Carbohydrates: 58g;
Sugar: 17g; Fiber: 7g; Fat: 8g;
Saturated Fat: 4g; Protein: 8g;
Sodium: 133mg

1 Grease a 6-quart slow cooker with plain vegetable oil.

2 In the slow cooker, mix the steel-cut oats, carrot, and pineapple.

3 In a medium bowl, mix the almond milk, water, coconut oil, honey, vanilla, salt, and cinnamon. Mix until well combined. Pour this mixture into the slow cooker.

4 Cover and cook on low for 6 to 8 hours, or until the oatmeal is tender and the edges start to brown.

VARIATION TIP
For an indulgent treat, serve this oatmeal with a creamy hard sauce. Mix 4 tablespoons softened cream cheese with about 2 tablespoons coconut sugar and 3 table-spoons Greek yogurt. Put a spoonful onto each serving of the hot oatmeal.

PUMPKIN PIE BAKED OATMEAL

SERVES 10 // PREP TIME: 15 MINUTES // COOK TIME: 6 TO 8 HOURS

Adding solid pack canned pumpkin to oatmeal makes it taste like pumpkin pie! Some granola sprinkled over the top adds a bit of crunch. You can leave the nuts out of this recipe if you'd like and choose a nut-free granola.

3 cups steel-cut oats

1 (16-ounce) can solid pack pumpkin

2 cups canned coconut milk

4 cups water

¼ cup honey

2 teaspoons vanilla extract

¼ teaspoon salt

1 teaspoon ground cinnamon

½ teaspoon ground ginger

1 cup granola

D Dairy-Free

G Gluten-Free

V Vegetarian

NUTRITION INFORMATION
Calories: 278; Carbohydrates: 51g; Sugar: 13g; Fiber: 7g; Fat: 5g; Saturated Fat: 2g; Protein: 7g; Sodium: 77mg

1 Grease a 6-quart slow cooker with plain vegetable oil.

2 Put the oats into the slow cooker.

3 In a medium bowl, mix the canned pumpkin and coconut milk with a wire whisk until blended. Then stir in the water, honey, vanilla, salt, cinnamon, and ginger. Mix until well combined. Pour this mixture into the slow cooker over the oats and stir. Top with the granola.

4 Cover and cook on low for 6 to 8 hours, or until the oatmeal is tender and the edges start to brown.

INGREDIENT TIP
Do not use pumpkin puree or pumpkin pie filling in this recipe, because they contain sweeteners, stabilizers, and emulsifiers that you don't want on the eating clean plan. Use plain solid pack pumpkin with one ingredient on the label: pumpkin.

FRENCH VEGETABLE OMELET

SERVES 6 // PREP TIME: 20 MINUTES // COOK TIME: 3 TO 4 HOURS

Lots of vegetables and herbs make this omelet so good. It's not as soft and tender as a traditional French omelet, but the ingredients add a French accent. Serve it with orange juice, coffee, and some fresh fruit.

12 eggs, beaten

⅓ cup 2% milk

½ teaspoon dried thyme leaves

½ teaspoon dried tarragon leaves

¼ teaspoon salt

1 cup chopped fresh asparagus

1 yellow bell pepper, stemmed, seeded, and chopped

1 small zucchini, peeled and diced

2 shallots, peeled and minced

½ cup grated Parmesan cheese

G Gluten-Free

N Nut-Free

V Vegetarian

NUTRITION INFORMATION
Calories: 205; Carbohydrates: 7g;
Sugar: 3g; Fiber: 1g; Fat: 12g;
Saturated Fat: 5g; Protein: 17g;
Sodium: 471mg

1 Grease the inside of a 6-quart slow cooker with plain vegetable oil.

2 In a large bowl, mix the eggs, milk, thyme, tarragon, and salt, and mix well with an eggbeater or wire whisk until well combined.

3 Add the asparagus, bell pepper, zucchini, and shallots. Pour into the slow cooker.

4 Cover and cook on low for 3 to 4 hours, or until the eggs are set.

5 Sprinkle with the Parmesan cheese; cover and cook for another 5 to 10 minutes or until the cheese starts to melt.

SUBSTITUTION TIP
Other vegetables such as broccoli florets, cauliflower florets, or yellow summer squash would be delicious in this omelet. You could also use other dried herbs, such as basil, chervil, or marjoram.

EGG AND WILD RICE CASSEROLE

SERVES 6 // PREP TIME: 20 MINUTES // COOK TIME: 5 TO 7 HOURS

Wild rice makes a great substitute for bread or potatoes in this breakfast casserole. You can use leftover wild rice from the recipe on page 41 or cook it yourself. Lots of vegetables make this recipe colorful and healthy.

3 cups plain cooked wild rice or Herbed Wild Rice (page 41)

2 cups sliced mushrooms

1 red bell pepper, stemmed, seeded, and chopped

1 onion, minced

2 garlic cloves, minced

11 eggs

1 teaspoon dried thyme leaves

¼ teaspoon salt

1½ cups shredded Swiss cheese

G Gluten-Free

N Nut-Free

V Vegetarian

NUTRITION INFORMATION*
Calories: 360; Carbohydrates: 25g; Sugar: 3g; Fiber: 3g; Fat: 17g; Saturated Fat: 8g; Protein: 24g; Sodium: 490mg

* Nutrition information uses plain cooked wild rice.

1 In a 6-quart slow cooker, layer the wild rice, mushrooms, bell pepper, onion, and garlic.

2 In a large bowl, beat the eggs with the thyme and salt. Pour into the slow cooker. Top with the cheese.

3 Cover and cook on low for 5 to 7 hours, or until a food thermometer registers 165°F and the casserole is set.

INGREDIENT TIP
You'll need ¾ cup of uncooked wild rice to yield 3 cups cooked. Mix the rice with 2 cups of water in a saucepan. Cover and simmer for 30 to 40 minutes, or until the rice is tender. Drain if necessary.

BANANA BREAD OATMEAL

SERVES 8 // PREP TIME: 20 MINUTES // COOK TIME: 7 TO 8 HOURS

Oatmeal is a healthy and delicious breakfast recipe, but it can be bland and kind of boring. This recipe adds the flavors of banana bread, a family favorite, to this morning staple. Mashed bananas, cinnamon, nutmeg, and some coconut milk make this recipe creamy and delicious.

4 cups coconut milk

4 cups water

2 cups steel cut oats

3 ripe bananas, peeled and mashed

⅓ cup coconut sugar

2 teaspoons ground cinnamon

½ teaspoon ground nutmeg

2 teaspoons vanilla extract

1 cup chopped pecans

1 Combine the coconut milk and water in a 6-quart slow cooker. Add the steel cut oats, bananas, coconut sugar, cinnamon, nutmeg, vanilla, and pecans.

2 Cover and cook on low for 7 to 8 hours or until the oats are very tender. Stir well before serving.

SUBSTITUTION TIP:
If bananas aren't your thing, you can substitute 1½ cups of applesauce or pureed pear for the mashed bananas in this recipe. If you do, reduce the water to 3 cups, since those ingredients have more liquid than the mashed bananas.

Ⓓ Dairy-Free

Ⓖ Gluten-Free

Ⓥ Vegan

NUTRITION INFORMATION
Calories: 545; Carbohydrates: 50g;
Sugar: 17g; Fiber: 7g; Fat: 35g;
Saturated Fat: 24g; Protein: 9g;
Sodium: 21mg

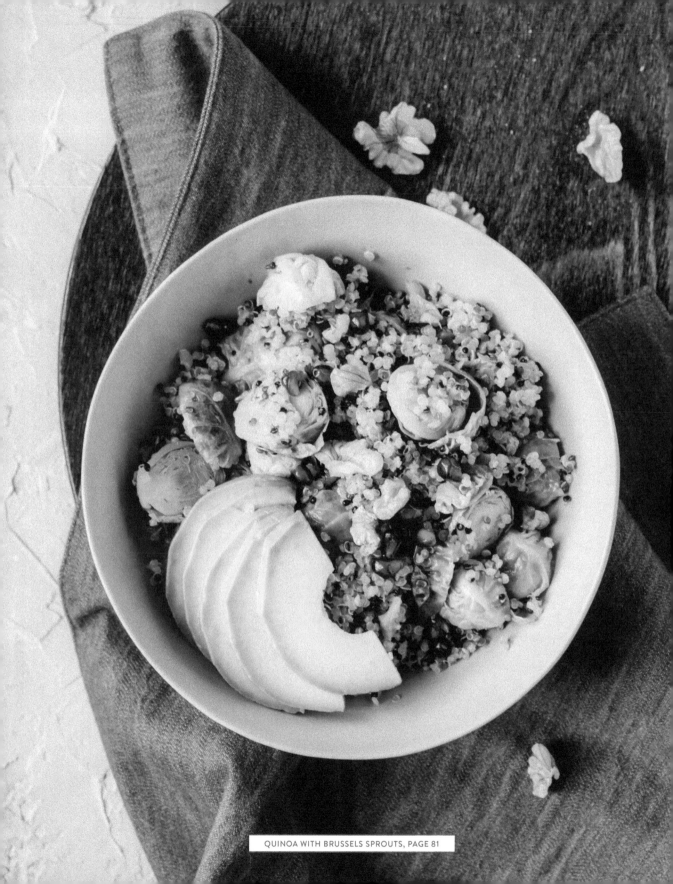

QUINOA WITH BRUSSELS SPROUTS, PAGE 81

CHAPTER FIVE

SIDES

MIXED POTATO GRATIN

SERVES 8 // PREP TIME: 20 MINUTES // COOK TIME: 7 TO 9 HOURS

Any recipe labeled gratin usually means "with cheese." This recipe mixes Yukon Gold and sweet potatoes for added color and nutrition. Just a bit of cheese is used for flavor and texture. This is a great dish to serve alongside a roasted chicken or some homemade meatloaf.

6 Yukon Gold potatoes, thinly sliced

3 sweet potatoes, peeled and thinly sliced

2 onions, thinly sliced

4 garlic cloves, minced

3 tablespoons whole-wheat flour

4 cups 2% milk, divided

1½ cups Roasted Vegetable Broth (page 30)

3 tablespoons melted butter

1 teaspoon dried thyme leaves

1½ cups shredded Havarti cheese

N Nut-Free

V Vegetarian

NUTRITION INFORMATION
Calories: 415; Carbohydrates: 42g; Sugar: 10g; Fiber: 3g; Fat: 22g; Saturated Fat: 13g; Protein: 17g; Sodium: 431mg

1 Grease a 6-quart slow cooker with plain vegetable oil.

2 In the slow cooker, layer the potatoes, onions, and garlic.

3 In a large bowl, mix the flour with ½ cup of the milk until well combined. Gradually add the remaining milk, stirring with a wire whisk to avoid lumps. Stir in the vegetable broth, melted butter, and thyme leaves.

4 Pour the milk mixture over the potatoes in the slow cooker and top with the cheese.

5 Cover and cook on low for 7 to 9 hours, or until the potatoes are tender when pierced with a fork.

VARIATION TIP
Leftovers of this recipe are great mixed with cooked chopped chicken or beef. Just mix together, then put into a casserole dish and bake until hot and bubbly.

ROASTED ROOT VEGETABLES

SERVES 8 // PREP TIME: 20 MINUTES // COOK TIME: 6 TO 8 HOURS

Root vegetables cook so beautifully in the slow cooker. And they are so good for you! Potatoes, carrots, sweet potatoes, and parsnips are full of fiber, vitamin C, and the B complex. They become tender and sweet when cooked this way and are the perfect side dish for a roasted chicken.

6 carrots, cut into
1-inch chunks

2 yellow onions, each cut into
8 wedges

2 sweet potatoes, peeled and
cut into chunks

6 Yukon Gold potatoes, cut
into chunks

8 whole garlic cloves, peeled

4 parsnips, peeled and cut
into chunks

3 tablespoons olive oil

1 teaspoon dried thyme leaves

½ teaspoon salt

⅛ teaspoon freshly ground
black pepper

In a 6-quart slow cooker, mix all of the ingredients. Cover and cook on low for 6 to 8 hours, or until the vegetables are tender.

SUBSTITUTION TIP
You can use other root vegetables in this easy recipe. Try adding some beets or peeled rutabagas. Red onion would be a nice substitute for the yellow onions too.

D Dairy-Free

G Gluten-Free

N Nut-Free

V Vegan

NUTRITION INFORMATION
Calories: 214; Carbohydrates: 40g;
Sugar: 7g; Fiber: 6g; Fat: 5g;
Saturated Fat: 1g; Protein: 4g;
Sodium: 201mg

STEWED HERBED FRUIT

SERVES 12 // PREP TIME: 15 MINUTES // COOK TIME: 6 TO 8 HOURS

Stewed fruit is made of dried fruits that are cooked in water and seasonings until they are tender. They are usually made with cinnamon and vanilla, but this recipe adds herbs instead for a more interesting taste. Serve this with Greek yogurt for breakfast or add it to hot cooked cereal.

2 cups dried apricots

2 cups prunes

2 cups dried unsulfured pears

2 cups dried apples

1 cup dried cranberries

¼ cup honey

6 cups water

1 teaspoon dried thyme leaves

1 teaspoon dried basil leaves

D Dairy-Free

G Gluten-Free

N Nut-Free

V Vegetarian

NUTRITION INFORMATION
Calories: 242; Carbohydrates: 61g;
Sugar: 43g; Fiber: 9g; Fat: 0g;
Saturated Fat: 0g; Protein: 2g;
Sodium: 11mg

1 In a 6-quart slow cooker, mix all of the ingredients. Cover and cook on low for 6 to 8 hours, or until the fruits have absorbed the liquid and are tender.

2 Store in the refrigerator up to 1 week. You can freeze the fruit in 1-cup portions for longer storage.

INGREDIENT TIP
Dried fruits are high in sugar, but when they are rehydrated, the sugar content decreases. These foods have a lot of fiber and are high in vitamin C. And remember that this sugar is natural sugar, not "added sugar."

ROASTED SQUASH PURÉE

SERVES 8 // PREP TIME: 20 MINUTES // COOK TIME: 6 TO 7 HOURS

A combination of two kinds of winter squash makes an interesting side dish. Winter squashes have thick skins, are quite hard, and can be stored for a long time. Peel them, remove the seeds, and cut them into cubes so they will cook evenly in the slow cooker.

1 (3-pound) butternut squash, peeled, seeded, and cut into 1-inch pieces

3 (1-pound) acorn squash, peeled, seeded, and cut into 1-inch pieces

2 onions, chopped

3 garlic cloves, minced

2 tablespoons olive oil

1 teaspoon dried marjoram leaves

½ teaspoon salt

⅛ teaspoon freshly ground black pepper

1 In a 6-quart slow cooker, mix all of the ingredients. Cover and cook on low for 6 to 7 hours, or until the squash is tender when pierced with a fork.

2 Use a potato masher to mash the squash right in the slow cooker.

VARIATION TIP
You can add some grated cheese to this recipe to make it more savory, or use cinnamon and cardamom in place of the marjoram for a sweeter version. If you use cinnamon and cardamom, add a couple of tablespoons of honey to the squash.

D Dairy-Free
G Gluten-Free
N Nut-Free
V Vegan

NUTRITION INFORMATION
Calories: 175; Carbohydrates: 38g;
Sugar: 1g; Fiber: 3g; Fat: 4g;
Saturated Fat: 1g; Protein: 3g;
Sodium: 149mg

HARVARD BEETS AND ONIONS

SERVES 8 // PREP TIME: 20 MINUTES // COOK TIME: 5 TO 7 HOURS

No one really knows how this recipe got its name. It's true that Harvard's school color is crimson, but the recipe wasn't invented there. No matter—if you love beets, this is a delicious recipe with a sweet and sour flavor. And red onions add another layer of flavor.

10 medium beets, peeled and sliced

3 red onions, chopped

4 garlic cloves, minced

⅓ cup honey

⅓ cup lemon juice

1 cup water

2 tablespoons melted coconut oil

3 tablespoons cornstarch

½ teaspoon salt

D Dairy-Free
G Gluten-Free
V Vegetarian

NUTRITION INFORMATION
Calories: 140; Carbohydrates: 27g;
Sugar: 19g; Fiber: 3g; Fat: 4g;
Saturated Fat: 3g; Protein: 2g;
Sodium: 218mg

1 In a 6-quart slow cooker, mix the beets, onions, and garlic.

2 In a medium bowl, mix the honey, lemon juice, water, coconut oil, cornstarch, and salt until well combined. Pour this mixture over the beets.

3 Cover and cook on low for 5 to 7 hours, or until the beets are tender and the sauce has thickened.

INGREDIENT TIP
Beet juice stains just about everything. Use gloves when you prepare them, and put newspaper or lots of paper towels over the work surface. You can use 3 to 4 cans of prepared sliced beets for this recipe if you'd like; cook for 3 to 4 hours on low.

HERBED LEAFY GREENS AND ONIONS

SERVES 8 // PREP TIME: 20 MINUTES // COOK TIME: 3 TO 4 HOURS

Leafy greens such as Swiss chard, collard greens, and kale are so good for you. They are packed full of fiber, vitamin C, vitamin A, potassium, and magnesium. When cooked with onions and herbs, they become tender, sweet, and flavorful.

2 bunches Swiss chard, washed and cut into large pieces

2 bunches collard greens, washed and cut into large pieces

2 bunches kale, washed and cut into large pieces

3 onions, chopped

1½ cups Roasted Vegetable Broth (page 30)

¼ cup honey

2 tablespoons lemon juice

1 teaspoon dried marjoram

1 teaspoon dried basil

¼ teaspoon salt

1 In a 6-quart slow cooker, mix the Swiss chard, collard greens, kale, and onions.

2 In a medium bowl, mix the vegetable broth, honey, lemon juice, marjoram, basil, and salt. Pour into the slow cooker.

3 Cover and cook on low for 3 to 4 hours, or until the greens are very tender.

INGREDIENT TIP
Swiss chard is made up of leaves and a stalk. It comes in green, red, or rainbow colors. Separate the stalk from the leaves. Cut the leaves into large pieces and the stalks into 2-inch pieces. Both are edible and delicious.

D Dairy-Free
G Gluten-Free
N Nut-Free
V Vegetarian

NUTRITION INFORMATION
Calories: 80; Carbohydrates: 19g;
Sugar: 11g; Fiber: 3g; Fat: 0g;
Saturated Fat: 0g; Protein: 3g;
Sodium: 118mg

CARAMELIZED ONIONS AND GARLIC

SERVES 12 // PREP TIME: 20 MINUTES // COOK TIME: 8 TO 10 HOURS

Caramelized onions are not only a fabulous side dish, but also a great seasoning. Add them to chicken, salmon, soups, stews, and casseroles. The deep golden brown onions are very sweet because the slow cooker caramelizes the sugar in this root vegetable, while the strong sulfurous compounds evaporate.

10 large yellow onions, peeled and sliced

20 garlic cloves, peeled

¼ cup olive oil

¼ teaspoon salt

2 tablespoons balsamic vinegar

1 teaspoon dried thyme leaves

Ⓓ Dairy-Free
Ⓖ Gluten-Free
Ⓝ Nut-Free
Ⓥ Vegetarian

NUTRITION INFORMATION
Calories: 109; Carbohydrates: 16g;
Sugar: 9g; Fiber: 3g; Fat: 4g;
Saturated Fat: 1g; Protein: 2g;
Sodium: 56mg

1 In a 6-quart slow cooker, mix all of the ingredients. Cover and cook on low for 8 to 10 hours, stirring once or twice if you have the time.

2 Refrigerate the onions up to 1 week, or divide them into 1-cup portions and freeze up to 3 months.

SUBSTITUTION TIP
Try using red onions in place of the yellow onions. These colorful onions are sweeter than yellow onions and make a great condiment or pizza topping.

TEX-MEX KALE WITH GARLIC

SERVES 8 // PREP TIME: 20 MINUTES // COOK TIME: 4 TO 5 HOURS

Kale is a super dark green leafy vegetable and has a bitter edge, but it becomes sweeter in the slow cooker. Add some Tex-Mex flavorings to make this a wonderful side dish.

4 bunches kale, washed, stemmed, and cut into large pieces

2 onions, chopped

8 garlic cloves, minced

2 jalapeño peppers, minced

4 large tomatoes, seeded and chopped

1 tablespoon chili powder

½ teaspoon salt

⅛ teaspoon freshly ground black pepper

1 In a 6-quart slow cooker, mix the kale, onions, garlic, jalapeño peppers, and tomatoes.

2 Sprinkle with the chili powder, salt, and pepper, and stir to mix.

3 Cover and cook on low for 4 to 5 hours, or until the kale is wilted and tender.

INGREDIENT TIP
There are several kinds of kale, including lacinato (also called dinosaur kale), cavolo nero, curly kale, and red Russian kale. The name doesn't really matter; they are all delicious and good for you, and they all look a bit different. Choose the type that appeals to you.

D Dairy-Free
G Gluten-Free
N Nut-Free
V Vegan

NUTRITION INFORMATION
Calories: 52; Carbohydrates: 11g; Sugar: 5g; Fiber: 3g Fat: 1g; Saturated Fat: 0g; Protein: 3g; Sodium: 223mg

HERBED SMASHED POTATOES WITH GARLIC

SERVES 6 // PREP TIME: 20 MINUTES // COOK TIME: 5 TO 6 HOURS

Potatoes cook to perfection in the slow cooker. The small potatoes used in this recipe can be red potatoes, creamer potatoes, or small Yukon Gold potatoes. They are smashed, not mashed, for a slightly chunky texture. The peels are left on the potatoes for more texture and nutrition. Serve this dish with a grilled steak or roast chicken.

3½ pounds red or creamer potatoes, rinsed

2 onions, minced

12 garlic cloves, peeled and sliced

½ cup Roasted Vegetable Broth (page 30)

3 tablespoons olive oil

1 teaspoon dried thyme leaves

1 teaspoon dried dill leaves

½ teaspoon salt

⅓ cup grated Parmesan cheese

1 In a 6-quart slow cooker, mix the potatoes, onions, garlic, vegetable broth, olive oil, thyme, dill, and salt. Cover and cook on low for 5 to 6 hours, or until the potatoes are tender.

2 Using a potato masher, mash the potatoes in the slow cooker, leaving some chunky pieces. Stir in the Parmesan cheese and serve.

INGREDIENT TIP
New, red, or creamer potatoes are usually very clean and don't need much scrubbing. Rinse the potatoes, gently rubbing off any dirt that may be on them, being careful not to tear the delicate skin.

G Gluten-Free

N Nut-Free

V Vegetarian

NUTRITION INFORMATION
Calories: 321; Carbohydrates: 48g;
Sugar: 8g; Fiber: 7g; Fat: 10g;
Saturated Fat: 3g; Protein: 10g;
Sodium: 439mg

SPICY REFRIED BEANS

SERVES 8 // PREP TIME: 10 MINUTES // COOK TIME: 9 HOURS

"Refried" beans are not actually fried two times. They are first cooked, then fried in fat. But you can make refried beans without frying! Just mash them with a potato masher and mix in some healthy fat. This classic Mexican recipe is full of flavor and nutrition.

4 cups dried pinto beans, rinsed and drained

2 onions, minced

4 garlic cloves, minced

1 jalapeño pepper, minced

1 teaspoon dried oregano leaves

1 teaspoon salt

9 cups Roasted Vegetable Broth (page 30)

⅓ cup olive oil

(D) Dairy-Free
(G) Gluten-Free
(N) Nut-Free
(V) Vegetarian

NUTRITION INFORMATION
Calories: 444; Carbohydrates: 66g; Sugar: 4g; Fiber: 15g; Fat: 10g; Saturated Fat: 1g; Protein: 21g; Sodium: 469mg

1 In a 6-quart slow cooker, mix the beans, onions, garlic, jalapeño pepper, oregano, salt, and vegetable broth. Cover and cook on low for 8 hours, or until the beans have absorbed most of the liquid and are tender.

2 Remove the cover from the slow cooker and add the olive oil. Use a potato masher to mash the beans right in the slow cooker.

3 Cover and cook on low for another 30 to 40 minutes, then serve. If the beans aren't thick enough, remove the cover and cook on high for 40 to 50 minutes longer, stirring occasionally.

VARIATION TIP
You can serve these refried beans as a side dish, or you can use them to make burritos, tacos, or enchiladas.

ORANGE HERBED CAULIFLOWER

SERVES 8 // PREP TIME: 20 MINUTES // COOK TIME: 4 HOURS

Cauliflower is a cruciferous vegetable. That means it is part of the family that includes cabbage and broccoli. Cauliflower is a good source of vitamins C and K, folate and fiber. It has a mild taste and tender texture when cooked in the slow cooker.

2 heads cauliflower, rinsed and cut into florets

2 onions, chopped

½ cup orange juice

1 teaspoon grated orange zest

1 teaspoon dried thyme leaves

½ teaspoon dried basil leaves

½ teaspoon salt

D Dairy-Free
G Gluten-Free
N Nut-Free
V Vegan

1 In a 6-quart slow cooker, mix the cauliflower and onions. Top with the orange juice and orange zest, and drizzle with the thyme, basil, and salt.

2 Cover and cook on low for 4 hours, or until the cauliflower is tender when pierced with a fork.

VARIATION TIP
You can mash the cauliflower when it is tender and serve it as a substitute for mashed potatoes. Add a few table-spoons of olive oil to the cauliflower before you mash it.

NUTRITION INFORMATION
Calories: 75; Carbohydrates: 16g;
Sugar: 8g; Fiber: 5g; Fat: 0g;
Saturated Fat: 0g; Protein: 5g;
Sodium: 212mg

MUSHROOM RISOTTO

SERVES 8 // PREP TIME: 20 MINUTES // COOK TIME: 3 ½ TO 4 ½ HOURS

Risotto makes a fabulous side dish for any meal. Making risotto usually requires lots of attention while it's cooking; you must stir the rice almost constantly while adding broth. Using the slow cooker to make this dish is a huge time-saver.

8 ounces button mushrooms, sliced

8 ounces cremini mushrooms, sliced

8 ounces shiitake mushrooms, stems removed and sliced

2 onions, chopped

5 garlic cloves, minced

2 cups short-grain brown rice

1 teaspoon dried marjoram leaves

6 cups Roasted Vegetable Broth (page 30)

3 tablespoons unsalted butter

½ cup grated Parmesan cheese

1 In a 6-quart slow cooker, mix the mushrooms, onions, garlic, rice, marjoram, and vegetable broth.

2 Cover and cook on low for 3 to 4 hours, or until the rice is tender.

3 Stir in the butter and cheese. Cover and let cook on low for 20 minutes, then serve.

INGREDIENT TIP
Cremini mushrooms are immature portabella mushrooms, those really big, deep brown mushrooms that are often stuffed in recipes. And shiitake mushrooms have a thinner cap and long stem. They are often sold dried, but you can find them fresh in some large grocery stores.

G Gluten-Free

N Nut-Free

V Vegetarian

NUTRITION INFORMATION
Calories: 331; Carbohydrates: 51g;
Sugar: 3g; Fiber: 5g; Fat: 10g;
Saturated Fat: 5g; Protein: 11g;
Sodium: 368mg

BARLEY-ROOT VEGETABLE GRATIN

SERVES 8 // PREP TIME: 20 MINUTES // COOK TIME: 7 TO 9 HOURS

This combination of barley with root vegetables, cheese, and vegetable broth is a real treat. The root veggies sweeten as they slowly cook, and the barley gets tender and has a nutty taste. You could serve this as a vegetarian main dish.

2 cups hulled barley

2 onions, chopped

5 garlic cloves, minced

3 large carrots, peeled and sliced

2 sweet potatoes, peeled and cubed

4 Yukon Gold potatoes, cubed

7 cups Roasted Vegetable Broth (page 30)

1 teaspoon dried tarragon leaves

½ cup grated Parmesan cheese

1 In a 6-quart slow cooker, mix the barley, onions, garlic, carrots, sweet potatoes, and Yukon Gold potatoes. Add the vegetable broth and tarragon leaves.

2 Cover and cook on low for 7 to 9 hours, or until the barley is tender and the vegetables are tender too.

3 Stir in the cheese and serve.

VARIATION TIP
Stir in another kind of cheese in place of the Parmesan if you'd like. You will have to add more, simply because Parmesan has such a strong taste that not much is needed. Add 1½ to 2 cups of shredded Swiss, Havarti, Colby, or Cheddar.

N Nut-Free

V Vegetarian

NUTRITION INFORMATION
Calories: 356; Carbohydrates: 64g;
Sugar: 6g; Fiber: 12g; Fat: 5g;
Saturated Fat: 2g; Protein: 13g;
Sodium: 424mg

THAI ROASTED VEGGIES

SERVES 8 // PREP TIME: 20 MINUTES // COOK TIME: 6 TO 8 HOURS

The ingredients used in Thai cooking are coconut milk, curry paste, fish sauce (which is really high in sodium), limes, hot peppers, and ginger. Some of these ingredients are added to root vegetables that slowly roast in the slow cooker. Thai ingredients add some nice heat and spice to ordinary veggies.

4 large carrots, peeled and cut into chunks

2 onions, peeled and sliced

6 garlic cloves, peeled and sliced

2 parsnips, peeled and sliced

2 jalapeño peppers, minced

½ cup Roasted Vegetable Broth (page 30)

⅓ cup canned coconut milk

3 tablespoons lime juice

2 tablespoons grated fresh ginger root

2 teaspoons curry powder

1 In a 6-quart slow cooker, mix the carrots, onions, garlic, parsnips, and jalapeño peppers.

2 In a small bowl, mix the vegetable broth, coconut milk, lime juice, ginger root, and curry powder until well blended. Pour this mixture into the slow cooker.

3 Cover and cook on low for 6 to 8 hours, or until the vegetables are tender when pierced with a fork.

INGREDIENT TIP
Curry powder is a blend of many spices, including cinnamon, cumin, coriander, turmeric, and mustard. You can buy good-quality curry powder at most grocery stores, or you can make your own by combining these ingredients.

D Dairy-Free
G Gluten-Free
V Vegan

NUTRITION INFORMATION
Calories: 69; Carbohydrates: 13g; Sugar: 6g; Fiber: 3g; Fat: 3g; Saturated Fat: 3g; Protein: 1g; Sodium: 95mg

WHEAT BERRY–CRANBERRY PILAF

Wheat berries, also called groats, are whole grains of wheat that are missing only the hull. This wonderful whole grain cooks up tender and slightly chewy, with a sweet and nutty flavor. Mixed with cranberries and some mild cheese, it makes a wonderful pilaf.

3 cups wheat berries, rinsed and drained

2 leeks, peeled, rinsed, and chopped

7 cups Roasted Vegetable Broth (page 30)

2 tablespoons lemon juice

1½ cups dried cranberries

1 teaspoon dried thyme leaves

¼ teaspoon salt

1 cup chopped pecans

1½ cups shredded baby Swiss cheese

 Vegetarian

1 In a 6-quart slow cooker, mix the wheat berries, leeks, vegetable broth, lemon juice, cranberries, thyme, and salt. Cover and cook on low for 8 to 10 hours, or until the wheat berries are tender, but still slightly chewy.

2 Add the pecans and cheese. Cover and let stand for 10 minutes, then serve.

INGREDIENT TIP

Leeks are a member of the onion family, but they are much milder than yellow or red onions. They can contain quite a bit of sand since they are grown in sandy soil. To clean them, cut the root off, then cut in half. Put them in a sink full of cold water and massage the leaves. The sand will drop to the bottom of the sink. Then drain and chop them.

NUTRITION INFORMATION
Calories: 407; Carbohydrates: 59g; Sugar: 14g; Fiber: 10g; Fat: 14g fat; Saturated Fat: 4g; Protein: 13g; Sodium: 129mg

QUINOA WITH BRUSSELS SPROUTS

SERVES 8 // PREP TIME: 20 MINUTES // COOK TIME: 5 TO 6 HOURS

This unusual combination of ingredients is beautiful and delicious. The freshness of pomegranate seeds and avocados complements the nutty quinoa and slightly bitter Brussels sprouts. You can serve it as a side dish or as a vegetarian main dish. Omit the walnuts if you are allergic to nuts.

2 cups quinoa, rinsed

1 onion, finely chopped

3 garlic cloves, minced

4 cups Roasted Vegetable Broth (page 30)

3 cups Brussels sprouts

1 teaspoon dried marjoram leaves

2 tablespoons lemon juice

2 avocados, peeled and sliced

½ cup pomegranate seeds

1 cup broken walnuts

1 In a 6-quart slow cooker, mix the quinoa, onion, garlic, vegetable broth, Brussels sprouts, marjoram, and lemon juice. Cover and cook on low for 5 to 6 hours, or until the quinoa is tender.

2 Top with the avocados, pomegranate seeds, and walnuts, and serve.

INGREDIENT TIP
To prepare Brussels sprouts, first rinse them under cool running water. Trim the root end to remove any discoloration, and remove any wilted or discolored outer leaves. Then just cut the little sprouts in half or quarters.

D Dairy-Free

G Gluten-Free

V Vegan

NUTRITION INFORMATION
Calories: 358; Carbohydrates: 42g;
Sugar: 6g; Fiber: 8g; Fat: 17g;
Saturated Fat: 1g; Protein: 10g;
Sodium: 83mg;

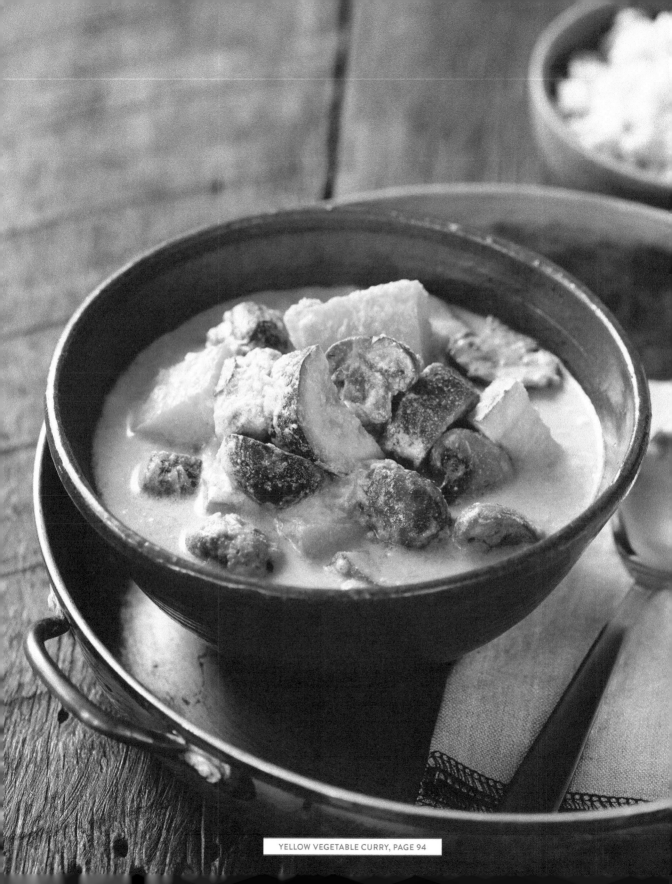
YELLOW VEGETABLE CURRY, PAGE 94

CHAPTER SIX

SOUPS AND STEWS

CHICKEN BARLEY STEW

SERVES 8 // PREP TIME: 20 MINUTES // COOK TIME: 8 TO 10 HOURS

This comforting and rich stew is the perfect thing to eat on a cold winter's night. The nutty barley complements the rich vegetables and tender chicken. Use chicken thighs because they take longer to cook than chicken breasts and won't overcook.

2 onions, chopped

4 garlic cloves, minced

4 large carrots, sliced

1¼ cups hulled barley

10 boneless, skinless chicken thighs, cut into 2-inch pieces

1½ cups frozen corn

8 cups Chicken Stock (page 26)

1 sprig fresh rosemary

1 teaspoon dried thyme leaves

2 cups baby spinach leaves

Ⓓ Dairy-Free

Ⓝ Nut-Free

NUTRITION INFORMATION
Calories: 430; Carbohydrates: 44g; Sugar: 11g; Fiber: 8g; Fat: 13g; Saturated Fat: 4g; Protein: 35g; Sodium: 501mg

1 In a 6-quart slow cooker, mix the onions, garlic, carrots, and barley. Top with the chicken and corn.

2 Pour the chicken stock over all and add the rosemary and thyme leaves.

3 Cover and cook on low for 8 to 10 hours, or until the chicken is cooked to 165°F and the barley is tender.

4 Remove and discard the rosemary stem. Stir in the spinach leaves. Cover and let stand for 5 minutes, then serve.

COOKING TIP
If you like a really thick stew, add a cornstarch slurry to this recipe. Mix 2 tablespoons cornstarch with ⅓ cup water and add to the slow cooker. Cover and cook on low for 10 minutes.

WILD RICE–VEGETABLE SOUP

SERVES 8 // PREP TIME: 20 MINUTES // COOK TIME: 7½ TO 9½ HOURS

This soup is a classic combination of vegetables and wild rice and is very delicious and so good for you. It cooks perfectly in the slow cooker while you are out of the house. Serve it with some toasted whole-wheat bread rubbed with garlic.

1½ cups wild rice, rinsed and drained

2 onions, chopped

1 leek, chopped

5 garlic cloves, sliced

2 cups sliced cremini mushrooms

4 carrots, peeled and sliced

2 cups frozen corn

8 cups Roasted Vegetable Broth (page 30)

1 teaspoon dried thyme leaves

2 cups chopped kale

1 In a 6-quart slow cooker, mix the wild rice, onions, leek, garlic, mushrooms, carrots, and corn.

2 Pour the vegetable broth over all and add the thyme leaves.

3 Cover and cook on low for 7 to 9 hours, or until the vegetables and wild rice are tender.

4 Stir in the kale. Cover and cook on low for another 20 minutes, or until the kale wilts.

VARIATION TIP
You can add just about any vegetable you'd like to this easy recipe. This is a vegan recipe, but you could add some chicken thighs if you'd like.

D Dairy-Free

G Gluten-Free

N Nut-Free

V Vegan

NUTRITION INFORMATION
Calories: 226; Carbohydrates: 46g;
Sugar: 8g; Fiber: 5g; Fat: 1g;
Saturated Fat: 0g; Protein: 7g;
Sodium: 172mg

HERBED CARROT-BARLEY SOUP

SERVES 8 // PREP TIME: 20 MINUTES
COOK TIME: 8 HOURS 15 MINUTES TO 9 HOURS 15 MINUTES

Did you know that carrot tops are edible and are very high in vitamin C, potassium, and calcium? Buy carrots with the tops and you can use the leafy greens in soups and stews. This recipe is warming and delicious and so healthy.

1½ cups hulled barley

1 bunch (about 6) large carrots, cut into 2-inch chunks and tops reserved

1 large celery root, peeled and cubed

2 onions, chopped

5 garlic cloves, minced

8 cups Roasted Vegetable Broth (page 30)

2 cups bottled unsweetened carrot juice

1 teaspoon dried dill weed

1 bay leaf

2 tablespoons freshly squeezed lemon juice

1 In a 6-quart slow cooker, mix the barley, carrots, celery root, onions, and garlic.

2 Add the vegetable broth, carrot juice, dill weed, and bay leaf.

3 Cover and cook on low for 8 to 9 hours, or until the barley and vegetables are tender. Remove and discard the bay leaf.

4 Chop the carrot tops and add 1 cup to the slow cooker. Add the lemon juice. Cover and cook on low for another 15 minutes.

INGREDIENT TIP
Celery root is also known as celeriac or celery knob and has a strong celery flavor. It's a very ugly vegetable and can be intimidating based on its looks alone. Just rinse it, peel it with a sharp knife, and cut it into cubes. It's delicious in stews and soups.

D Dairy-Free

N Nut-Free

V Vegan

NUTRITION INFORMATION
Calories: 220; Carbohydrates: 43g;
Sugar: 9g; Fiber: 9g; Fat: 1g;
Saturated Fat: 0g; Protein: 6g;
Sodium: 240mg

VEGETABLE WILD RICE CHILI

SERVES 8 // PREP TIME: 20 MINUTES // COOK TIME: 6 TO 7 HOURS

Wild rice is a great addition to a vegetarian chili recipe. It adds great flavor, textural interest, and a wonderful nutty taste. Canned beans are used in this recipe because, otherwise, the wild rice would overcook and get mushy in the time it takes dried beans to get tender.

1½ cups wild rice, rinsed and drained

2 onions, chopped

3 garlic cloves, minced

2 cups sliced cremini mushrooms

2 red bell peppers, stemmed, seeded, and chopped

2 (15-ounce) BPA-free cans no-salt-added black beans, drained and rinsed

1 tablespoon chili powder

½ teaspoon ground cumin

5 cups Roasted Vegetable Broth (page 30)

3 cups low-sodium tomato juice

In a 6-quart slow cooker, mix all of the ingredients. Cover and cook on low for 6 to 7 hours, or until the wild rice is tender.

RECIPE TIP
If you like really spicy food, you can add more ingredients to this chili. Add some minced jalapeño pepper, or add some crushed red pepper flakes or cayenne pepper.

D Dairy-Free
G Gluten-Free
N Nut-Free
V Vegan

NUTRITION INFORMATION
Calories: 288; Carbohydrates: 58g;
Sugar: 9g; Fiber: 10g; Fat: 5g;
Saturated Fat: 0g; Protein: 13g;
Sodium: 564mg

LENTIL-BARLEY SOUP

SERVES 8 // PREP TIME: 20 MINUTES
COOK TIME: 6 HOURS 15 MINUTES TO 7 HOURS 20 MINUTES

Lentils really add a lot to any soup recipe. They can be cooked until tender, or cooked for a very long time so they dissolve into the liquid, adding creaminess and texture to the soup. Pearl barley instead of hulled barley is used here so the lentils keep their shape.

2 onions, chopped

1 leek, chopped

4 garlic cloves, minced

4 large carrots, peeled and sliced

3 large tomatoes, seeded and chopped

1½ cups pearl barley

1½ cups puy lentils

12 cups Roasted Vegetable Broth (page 30)

1 teaspoon dried dill weed

2 cups chopped kale

D Dairy-Free
N Nut-Free
V Vegan

NUTRITION INFORMATION
Calories: 347; Carbohydrates: 66g;
Sugar: 10g; Fiber: 14g; Fat: 2g;
Saturated Fat: 0g; Protein: 16g;
Sodium: 250mg

1 In a 6-quart slow cooker, mix the onions, leek, garlic, carrots, tomatoes, barley, lentils, vegetable broth, and dill weed. Cover and cook on low for 6 to 7 hours, or until the barley and lentils are tender.

2 Stir in the kale; cover and cook on low for 15 to 20 minutes, or until the kale has wilted.

RECIPE TIP
This soup can be mild, as written, or you can spice it up with other ingredients. Try adding a minced habanero or serrano chili, or stir in some dried chili powder.

TEX-MEX BLACK BEAN AND CORN SOUP

SERVES 8 // PREP TIME: 20 MINUTES // COOK TIME: 8 TO 9 HOURS

Tex-Mex foods are a combination of classical Mexican foods and the flavors of Texas. These ingredients include beans, corn, chili peppers, tomatoes, onions, and garlic. All of them are mixed in this hearty stew that is delicious on a cold night.

3 cups dried black beans

2 onions, chopped

4 large tomatoes, seeded and chopped

6 garlic cloves, minced

2 jalapeño peppers, minced

3 cups frozen corn

2 tablespoons chili powder

1 teaspoon ground red chili

1 teaspoon ground cumin

11 cups Roasted Vegetable Broth (page 30)

In a 6-quart slow cooker, mix all of the ingredients. Cover and cook on low for 8 to 9 hours, or until the beans are tender.

INGREDIENT TIP
The heat in chili peppers is in the seeds and the membranes inside the pepper. If you like spicy food, leave them in when you prepare the peppers. But if you prefer a milder taste, remove and discard the seeds and membranes.

D Dairy-Free

G Gluten-Free

N Nut-Free

V Vegan

NUTRITION INFORMATION
Calories: 336; Carbohydrates: 65g;
Sugar: 13g; Fiber: 20g; Fat: 1g;
Saturated Fat: 0g; Protein: 18g;
Sodium: 229mg

CARAMELIZED ONION AND GARLIC BORSCHT

SERVES 8 // PREP TIME: 20 MINUTES
COOK TIME: 6 HOURS 15 MINUTES TO 7 HOURS 20 MINUTES

Borscht is a Russian recipe typically made of roasted beets that are puréed with chicken stock and served with sour cream. You can make this a vegetarian recipe simply by replacing the chicken stock with vegetable broth. If you don't have Caramelized Onions and Garlic (page 72), you can add 2 chopped onions and 8 cloves of sliced garlic to the slow cooker along with the beets and carrots.

8 large beets, peeled and cubed

2 cups Caramelized Onions and Garlic (page 72)

3 large carrots, peeled and chopped

8 cups Roasted Vegetable Broth (page 30)

5 tablespoons tomato paste (see tip on page 31)

1 bay leaf

1 teaspoon dried dill weed

1 cup sour cream

2 tablespoons cornstarch

G Gluten-Free

N Nut-Free

V Vegetarian

NUTRITION INFORMATION
Calories: 239; Carbohydrates: 31g; Sugar: 18g; Fiber: 6g; Fat: 8g; Saturated Fat: 4g; Protein: 10g; Sodium: 482mg

1 In a 6-quart slow cooker, mix the beets, onions, carrots, vegetable broth, tomato paste, bay leaf, and dill weed. Cover and cook on low for 6 to 7 hours, or until the beets and carrots are tender.

2 Remove and discard the bay leaf.

3 You can mash some of the vegetables right in the slow cooker if you'd like, or use an immersion blender.

4 Mix some of the liquid from the hot soup with the sour cream and cornstarch until well combined and stir into the soup.

5 Cover and cook on low for 15 to 20 minutes longer, or until the soup thickens.

VARIATION TIP
You can make this recipe with some cubed round steak and change the vegetable broth to beef broth for a more authentic version of borscht. Serve with more sour cream and some chopped fresh dill on top.

GINGERED PORK SWEET POTATO CHOWDER

SERVES 8 // PREP TIME: 20 MINUTES
COOK TIME: 6 HOURS 15 MINUTES TO 8 HOURS 20 MINUTES

A chowder is simply a soup that has been thickened with flour or cornstarch. It also usually means that milk or cream is added to the recipe. This easy dish combines pork with sweet potatoes and ginger to create a slightly spicy chowder that is rich and thick. Two kinds of ginger give it a kick.

1 (3-pound) pork loin, cut into 1½-inch cubes

2 leeks, chopped

4 large sweet potatoes, peeled and cubed

2 cups frozen corn

4 garlic cloves, minced

3 tablespoons grated fresh ginger root

1 teaspoon ground ginger

8 cups Roasted Vegetable Broth (page 30)

⅔ cup 2% milk

2 tablespoons cornstarch

1 In a 6-quart slow cooker, mix the pork, leeks, sweet potatoes, corn, garlic, ginger root, ground ginger, and vegetable broth. Cover and cook on low for 6 to 8 hours, or until the sweet potatoes are tender.

2 In a small bowl, whisk the milk and cornstarch until well blended. Stir this mixture into the slow cooker.

3 Cover and cook on low for 15 to 20 minutes longer, or until the chowder is thickened.

INGREDIENT TIP
The easiest way to peel fresh ginger root is to scrape it with a spoon. This knobby root is hard to chop or mince, so grate it on a cheese grater.

Ⓖ Gluten-Free

Ⓝ Nut-Free

NUTRITION INFORMATION
Calories: 382; Carbohydrates: 33g; Sugar: 11g; Fiber: 4g; Fat: 8g; Saturated Fat: 2g; Protein: 42g; Sodium: 414mg

BEEF-VEGETABLE CHILI

SERVES 8 // PREP TIME: 20 MINUTES // COOK TIME: 8 TO 10 HOURS

Classic chili is not made with beans; it contains just beef and vegetables, especially chili peppers. But for most people, chili means beans! You can use any dried bean you'd like in this easy recipe, from kidney beans to black beans. Serve it with sour cream, shredded cheese, and cubes of avocado.

2 cups dry beans, rinsed and drained

2½ pounds sirloin tip, cut into 2-inch cubes

2 onions, chopped

6 garlic cloves, minced

2 jalapeño peppers, minced

4 large tomatoes, seeded and chopped

11 cups Roasted Vegetable Broth (page 30)

1 (6-ounce) BPA-free can tomato paste (see tip on page 31)

2 tablespoons chili powder

1 teaspoon ground cumin

In a 6-quart slow cooker, mix all of the ingredients. Cover and cook on low for 8 to 10 hours, or until the beans are tender.

INGREDIENT TIP
Whenever you prepare any type of hot pepper, whether it's a jalapeño or a Scotch bonnet, never touch your face. The capsaicin in the chili will burn your eyes and lips. It's a good idea to use disposable gloves when handling chilies. Throw them away when you're done.

Ⓓ Dairy-Free
Ⓖ Gluten-Free
Ⓝ Nut-Free

NUTRITION INFORMATION
Calories: 459; Carbohydrates: 47g; Sugar: 10g; Fiber: 14g; Fat: 10g; Saturated Fat: 3g; Protein: 45g; Sodium: 290mg

MOROCCAN SIRLOIN SWEET POTATO STEW

SERVES 8 // PREP TIME: 20 MINUTES // COOK TIME: 7 TO 9 HOURS

The foods of Morocco include beef, couscous, dried fruits, olive oil, lemons, and spices. These are combined in this wonderfully rich and fragrant stew. The couscous, which is added at the end of the cooking time, thickens the liquid into a thick sauce.

2 pounds sirloin tip, cut into 2-inch pieces

2 onions, chopped

3 garlic cloves, minced

2 large sweet potatoes, peeled and cubed

⅔ cup chopped dried apricots

⅔ cup golden raisins

5 large tomatoes, seeded and chopped

9 cups Beef Stock (page 27)

2 teaspoons curry powder

1 cup whole-wheat couscous, cooked according to package directions

D Dairy-Free

N Nut-Free

NUTRITION INFORMATION
Calories: 383; Carbohydrates: 51g;
Sugar: 21g; Fiber: 7g; Fat: 7g;
Saturated Fat: 2g; Protein: 30g;
Sodium: 200mg

1   In a 6-quart slow cooker, mix the sirloin, onions, garlic, sweet potatoes, apricots, raisins, tomatoes, beef stock, and curry powder. Cover and cook on low for 7 to 9 hours, or until the sweet potatoes are tender.

2   Stir in the couscous. Cover and let stand for 5 to 10 minutes, or until the couscous has softened.

3   Stir the stew and serve.

INGREDIENT TIP
Couscous is not a grain, but rather a small pasta. It comes in two sizes. The first is very small and quick cooking. The larger form, also called Israeli couscous, is about the size of peppercorns. They have different cooking instructions; follow the directions on the package.

YELLOW VEGETABLE CURRY

SERVES 8 // PREP TIME: 20 MINUTES // COOK TIME: 6 TO 8 HOURS

This easy vegan recipe is perfect for dinner on a cold night. The colors are beautiful, and the combination of ingredients provides lots of nutrients, especially antioxidants and fiber. Use the amount of curry paste suited to your tastes.

2 onions, chopped

3 garlic cloves, minced

2 medium zucchini, cut into 1-inch slices

2 medium sweet potatoes, peeled and cut into chunks

3 cups broccoli florets

4 large carrots, peeled and cut into chunks

1 (8 ounce) package button mushrooms, sliced

2 red bell peppers, stemmed, seeded, and chopped

5 cups Roasted Vegetable Broth (page 30)

1 cup canned coconut milk

2 to 4 tablespoons yellow curry paste

1 In a 6-quart slow cooker, mix all the ingredients. Cover and cook on low for 6 to 8 hours, or until the vegetables are tender.

2 Serve in soup bowls over hot cooked brown rice, if you prefer.

INGREDIENT TIP
Curry paste is an intense condiment that adds great flavor and color to Indian dishes. It comes in several colors: Yellow is medium intensity, while red can be very hot and green is the mildest. Taste them and use the one you like best.

Ⓓ Dairy-Free

Ⓖ Gluten-Free

Ⓥ Vegan

NUTRITION INFORMATION
Calories: 161; Carbohydrates: 32g;
Sugar: 9g; Fiber: 6g; Fat: 6g;
Saturated Fat: 5g; Protein: 4g;
Sodium: 662mg

ROASTED TOMATO BISQUE

SERVES 8 // PREP TIME: 20 MINUTES // COOK TIME: 9 HOURS 10 MINUTES

In this easy recipe, tomatoes, onions, and garlic are roasted in the slow cooker until they start to brown. Then vegetable broth is added along with milk, and the whole thing is puréed right in the slow cooker.

3 pounds tomatoes, quartered

2 onions, chopped

2 shallots, minced

4 garlic cloves, minced

½ teaspoon salt

8 cups Roasted Vegetable Broth (page 30)

1 teaspoon dried dill weed

1 teaspoon honey

⅛ teaspoon freshly ground black pepper

1½ cups whole milk

G Gluten-Free

N Nut-Free

V Vegetarian

NUTRITION INFORMATION
Calories: 100; Carbohydrates: 17g; Sugar: 10g; Fiber: 2g; Fat: 2g; Saturated Fat: 1g; Protein: 4g; Sodium: 250mg

1 In a 6-quart slow cooker, mix the tomatoes, onions, shallots, garlic, and salt. Cover and cook on low for 8 hours.

2 Add the vegetable broth, dill weed, honey, and pepper to the slow cooker. Cover and cook on high for 1 hour. Add the milk and cook for 10 minutes longer.

3 Use an immersion blender or a potato masher to puree the soup to desired consistency.

SUBSTITUTION TIP
To make this a vegan recipe, omit the honey and use almond milk in place of the regular whole milk. Of course, this changes the recipe so it is no longer nut-free!

FRENCH CHICKEN–WILD RICE STEW

SERVES 8 // PREP TIME: 20 MINUTES // COOK TIME: 7 TO 9 HOURS

So what makes a recipe "French?" The ingredients it uses! Tomatoes, basil and other herbs, olive oil, garlic, and olives are all classic French ingredients. This rich and hearty stew also uses wild rice for a twist and some interesting texture.

1 cup wild rice, rinsed and drained

2 cups sliced cremini mushrooms

2 leeks, chopped

3 large carrots, sliced

3 garlic cloves, minced

10 boneless, skinless chicken thighs, cut into 2-inch pieces

8 cups Roasted Vegetable Broth (page 30)

2 (14-ounce) BPA-free cans diced tomatoes, undrained

½ cup sliced ripe olives

2 teaspoon dried herbes de Provence

In a 6-quart slow cooker, mix all of the ingredients. Cover and cook on low for 7 to 9 hours, or until the chicken is cooked to 165°F and the wild rice is tender.

INGREDIENT TIP
Herbes de Provence is a blend of several herbs, including rosemary, savory, thyme, marjoram, basil, oregano, and fennel. You can make your own blend if you can't find it in the store. Keep it in an airtight container in a cool, dark place.

D Dairy-Free
G Gluten-Free
N Nut-Free

NUTRITION INFORMATION
Calories: 363; Carbohydrates: 31g; Sugar: 5g; Fiber: 3g; Fat: 12g; Saturated Fat: 0g; Protein: 32g; Sodium: 470mg

PASTA PRIMAVERA STEW

SERVES 8 // PREP TIME: 20 MINUTES // COOK TIME: 6½ TO 7½ HOURS

Pasta primavera is simply pasta with vegetables in a tomato sauce. This recipe turns that dish into a healthy and warming soup. Lots of fresh vegetables make this recipe very colorful and healthy.

2 onions, chopped

5 garlic cloves, minced

2 cups sliced button mushrooms

2 cups sliced cremini mushrooms

2 cups chopped yellow summer squash

2 red bell peppers, stemmed, seeded, and chopped

6 large tomatoes, seeded and chopped

8 cups Roasted Vegetable Broth (page 30)

2 teaspoons dried Italian seasoning

1½ cups whole-wheat orzo pasta

D Dairy-Free

N Nut-Free

V Vegan

NUTRITION INFORMATION
Calories: 248; Carbohydrates: 48g;
Sugar: 10g; Fiber: 9g; Fat: 1g;
Saturated Fat: 0g; Protein: 11g;
Sodium: 462mg

1 In a 6-quart slow cooker, mix the onions, garlic, mushrooms, summer squash, bell peppers, tomatoes, vegetable broth, and Italian seasoning. Cover and cook on low for 6 to 7 hours, or until the vegetables are tender.

2 Add the pasta and stir. Cover and cook on low for another 20 to 30 minutes, or until the pasta is tender.

VARIATION TIP
Add some chopped cooked chicken or leftover cooked beef to this recipe if you'd like. Then top the soup with some grated Parmesan cheese before serving.

SALMON-VEGGIE CHOWDER

SERVES 8 // PREP TIME: 20 MINUTES // COOK TIME: 6 ½ TO 8 ½ HOURS

Salmon cooks well in the slow cooker, but it takes only about 30 minutes to cook on low. So the rest of this soup cooks for hours, and you add the salmon just before you're ready to eat. This colorful chowder is delicious and healthy.

6 medium Yukon Gold potatoes, cut into 2-inch pieces

4 large carrots, sliced

2 cups sliced cremini mushrooms

4 shallots, minced

3 garlic cloves, minced

8 cups Roasted Vegetable Broth (page 30) or Fish Stock (page 28)

2 teaspoons dried dill weed

2 pounds skinless salmon fillets

1 cup whole milk

1½ cups shredded Swiss cheese

1 In a 6-quart slow cooker, mix the potatoes, carrots, mushrooms, shallots, garlic, vegetable broth, and dill weed. Cover and cook on low for 6 to 8 hours, or until the vegetables are tender.

2 Add the salmon fillets to the slow cooker. Cover and cook on low for another 20 to 30 minutes, or until the salmon flakes when tested with a fork.

3 Stir the chowder to break up the salmon.

4 Add the milk and Swiss cheese and cover. Let the chowder stand 10 minutes to let the cheese melt. Stir the chowder and serve.

RECIPE TIP
If you'd like your chowder to be thicker, add 2 table-spoons cornstarch to the milk before you stir it into the slow cooker. Then cook the chowder for another 10 to 15 minutes until it's thickened.

G Gluten-Free

N Nut-Free

NUTRITION INFORMATION
Calories: 453; Carbohydrates: 31g; Sugar: 6g; Fiber: 3g; Fat: 20g; Saturated Fat: 7g; Protein: 34g; Sodium: 252mg

RATATOUILLE SOUP

SERVES 8 // PREP TIME: 20 MINUTES // COOK TIME: 7 TO 9 HOURS

Ratatouille is a vegetarian main dish composed of eggplant, tomatoes, garlic, and bell peppers. It is layered, baked, and topped with cheese. This recipe turns it into a colorful and rich soup full of great flavors.

2 tablespoons olive oil

2 onions, chopped

4 garlic cloves, minced

2 medium eggplant, peeled and chopped

2 red bell peppers, stemmed, seeded, and chopped

6 large tomatoes, seeded and chopped

6 cups Roasted Vegetable Broth (page 30)

2 teaspoons herbes de Provence

1½ cups shredded Swiss cheese

2 tablespoons cornstarch

G Gluten-Free

N Nut-Free

V Vegetarian

NUTRITION INFORMATION
Calories: 215; Carbohydrates: 23g; Sugar: 11g; Fiber: 8g; Fat: 10g; Saturated Fat: 4g; Protein: 9g; Sodium: 144mg

1 In a 6-quart slow cooker, mix the olive oil, onions, garlic, eggplant, bell peppers, tomatoes, vegetable broth, and herbes de Provence. Cover and cook on low for 7 to 9 hours, or until the vegetables are tender.

2 In a small bowl, toss the cheese with the cornstarch. Add the cheese mixture to the slow cooker. Cover and let stand for 10 minutes, then stir the soup and serve.

RECIPE TIP
Like all soups, this one freezes beautifully. Cool the soup down in shallow containers in the refrigerator, then transfer it to freezer-proof containers. Freeze up to 3 months. To use, thaw in the refrigerator overnight, then heat up the soup in a saucepan on the stove until it just comes to a simmer.

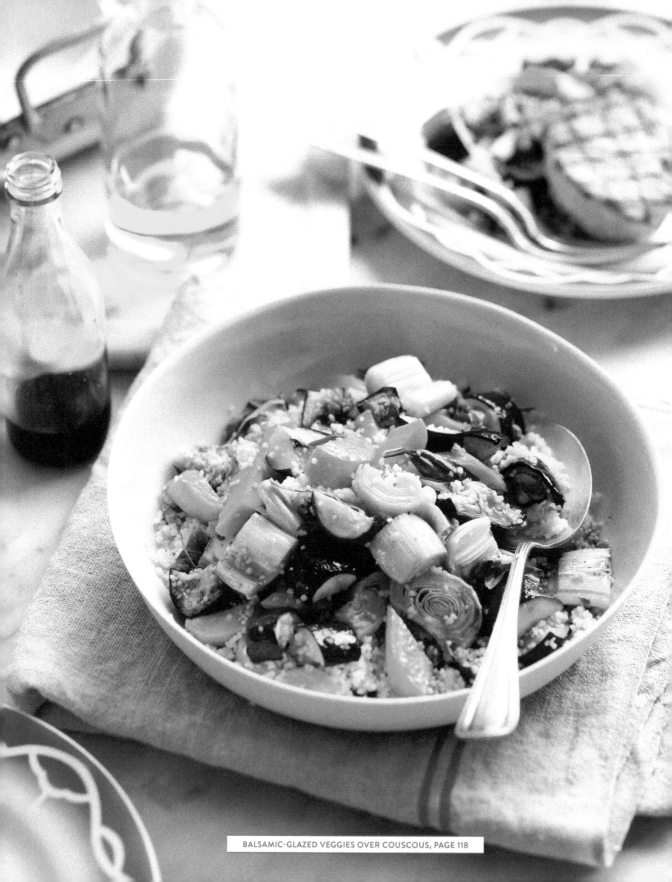

BALSAMIC-GLAZED VEGGIES OVER COUSCOUS, PAGE 118

CHAPTER SEVEN

VEGETABLES
AND MORE VEGETABLES

STUFFED TOMATOES

SERVES 6 // PREP TIME: 20 MINUTES // COOK TIME: 6 TO 7 HOURS

Flavorful and tender tomatoes are stuffed with a mixture of bread crumbs and vegetables, then cooked in the slow cooker. This rich-tasting recipe is full of vitamins and minerals and makes a great side dish or vegetarian main dish.

6 large tomatoes

1 red onion, finely chopped

1 yellow bell pepper, stemmed, seeded, and chopped

3 garlic cloves, minced

¾ cup low-sodium whole-wheat bread crumbs

1½ cups shredded Colby cheese

¼ cup finely chopped flat-leaf parsley

1 teaspoon dried thyme leaves

½ cup Roasted Vegetable Broth (page 30)

Ⓝ Nut-Free
Ⓥ Vegetarian

NUTRITION INFORMATION
Calories: 187; Carbohydrates: 22g; Sugar: 6g; Fiber: 4g; Fat: 7g; Saturated Fat: 4g; Protein: 9g; Sodium: 143mg

1 Cut the tops off the tomatoes. With a serrated spoon, core the tomatoes, reserving the pulp. Set the tomatoes aside.

2 In a medium bowl, mix the onion, bell pepper, garlic, bread crumbs, cheese, parsley, thyme, and reserved tomato pulp.

3 Stuff this mixture into the tomatoes, and place the tomatoes in a 6-quart slow cooker. Pour the vegetable broth into the bottom of the slow cooker.

4 Cover and cook on low for 6 to 7 hours, or until the tomatoes are tender.

VARIATION TIP
You can use this filling to stuff bell peppers as well. Use 8 bell peppers and substitute 3 chopped tomatoes for the bell pepper in this recipe.

CURRIED SQUASH

SERVES 8 // PREP TIME: 20 MINUTES // COOK TIME: 6 TO 7 HOURS

All types of winter squash make a fabulous slow cooker side dish. This recipe uses three kinds of squash for interest and nutrition. Serve it with a roasted chicken or a grilled steak.

1 large butternut squash, peeled, seeded, and cut into 1-inch pieces

3 acorn squash, peeled, seeded, and cut into 1-inch pieces

2 onions, finely chopped

5 garlic cloves, minced

1 tablespoon curry powder

⅓ cup freshly squeezed orange juice

½ teaspoon salt

In a 6-quart slow cooker, mix all of the ingredients. Cover and cook on low for 6 to 7 hours, or until the squash is tender when pierced with a fork.

VARIATION TIP
You can mash the squash in this recipe and serve it as a substitute for mashed potatoes. Use a potato masher or immersion blender to puree the squash right in the slow cooker.

D Dairy-Free
G Gluten-Free
N Nut-Free
V Vegan

NUTRITION INFORMATION
Calories: 88; Carbohydrates: 24g; Sugar: 4g; Fiber: 3g; Fat: 0g; Saturated Fat: 0g; Protein: 2g; Sodium: 169mg

HERBED SUCCOTASH

SERVES 10 // PREP TIME: 20 MINUTES // COOK TIME: 8 TO 9 HOURS

Succotash is a classic Southern recipe and is made of corn and lima beans. This combination is delicious, and this recipe is very easy to make.

2 cups dry lima beans, rinsed and drained

4 cups frozen corn

1 red onion, minced

4 large tomatoes, seeded and chopped

5 cups Roasted Vegetable Broth (page 30)

1 teaspoon dried thyme leaves

1 teaspoon dried basil leaves

1 bay leaf

In a 6-quart slow cooker, mix all of the ingredients. Cover and cook on low for 8 to 9 hours, or until the lima beans are tender. Remove and discard the bay leaf.

VARIATION TIP
You can substitute edamame, or soybeans, for the lima beans in this easy recipe. Prepare them just as you would the lima beans and continue with the recipe.

(D) Dairy-Free

(G) Gluten-Free

(N) Nut-Free

(V) Vegan

NUTRITION INFORMATION
Calories: 128; Carbohydrates: 27g; Sugar: 10g; Fiber: 6g; Fat: 1g; Saturated Fat: 0g; Protein: 6g; Sodium: 73mg

TEX-MEX SWEET POTATOES AND ONIONS

SERVES 8 // PREP TIME: 20 MINUTES // COOK TIME: 7 TO 8 HOURS

Most recipes using sweet potatoes use other sweet ingredients. But try combining that nutritional powerhouse with some spicy Tex-Mex flavors, and you have a side dish everyone will love. Serve this with meatloaf or a grilled steak.

5 large sweet potatoes, peeled and chopped

3 onions, chopped

5 garlic cloves, minced

2 jalapeño or habanero peppers, minced

2 tablespoons olive oil

⅓ cup Roasted Vegetable Broth (page 30)

1 tablespoon chili powder

1 teaspoon ground cumin

½ teaspoon salt

1 In a 6-quart slow cooker, mix all of the ingredients. Cover and cook on low for 7 to 8 hours.

2 Stir the mixture gently but thoroughly and serve.

INGREDIENT TIP
You can use other types of chilies in this recipe. Chipotle chilies in adobo sauce are wonderful and spicy, but be aware that that ingredient can contain a lot of salt: as much as 240 mg for 2 tablespoons. Scotch bonnet chilies are super spicy, or you can use poblano chilies, which are mild.

D Dairy-Free
G Gluten-Free
N Nut-Free
V Vegan

NUTRITION INFORMATION
Calories: 172; Carbohydrates: 30g;
Sugar: 8g; Fiber: 5g; Fat: 5g;
Saturated Fat: 1g; Protein: 3g;
Sodium: 275mg

ROASTED BELL PEPPERS

SERVES 8 // PREP TIME: 20 MINUTES // COOK TIME: 5 TO 6 HOURS

Roasted bell peppers are perfect to cook in the slow cooker. This sweet vegetable caramelizes in the low heat and adds a slightly smoky taste to a dish. You can serve these as a side dish or add them to fajitas or soups and stews.

8 to 10 bell peppers of different colors, stemmed, seeded, and halved

1 red onion, chopped

1 tablespoon olive oil

1 teaspoon dried thyme leaves

D Dairy-Free
G Gluten-Free
N Nut-Free
V Vegan

NUTRITION INFORMATION
Calories: 59; Carbohydrates: 9g;
Sugar: 5g; Fiber: 3g; Fat: 2g;
Saturated Fat: 0g; Protein: 2g;
Sodium: 6mg

1 In a 6-quart slow cooker, place the bell pepper. Do not overfill your slow cooker. Drizzle with the olive oil, and top with the red onion and thyme. Cover and cook on low for 5 to 6 hours, stirring once if you are home, until the peppers are very tender and slightly browned on the edges.

2 You can remove the bell pepper skins if you'd like when they are done; they will come off very easily.

RECIPE TIP
You can freeze roasted bell peppers, or any roasted vegetable for that matter. Cool in the fridge, then divide into 2-cup portions and freeze up to 3 months. When you want to use them, let them thaw overnight in the refrigerator, then use them in recipes or as an appetizer.

ROASTED CARROTS AND PARSNIPS

SERVES 8 // PREP TIME: 20 MINUTES // COOK TIME: 5 TO 7 HOURS

Parsnips are an underrated and unappreciated root vegetable that seems old-fashioned. But when roasted, they are tender and sweet. And they are high in fiber, magnesium, potassium, iron, and vitamins B, C, E, and K.

6 large carrots, peeled and cut into 2-inch pieces

5 large parsnips, peeled and cut into 2-inch pieces

2 red onions, chopped

4 garlic cloves, minced

2 tablespoons olive oil

1 tablespoon honey

½ teaspoon salt

In a 6-quart slow cooker, mix all of the ingredients and stir gently. Cover and cook on low for 5 to 7 hours, or until the vegetables are tender.

VARIATION TIP
You can puree this mixture and serve it as a side dish to roasted chicken, pork chops, or meatloaf. Use a potato masher or immersion blender until the texture is as smooth as you want.

D Dairy-Free
G Gluten-Free
N Nut-Free
V Vegetarian

NUTRITION INFORMATION
Calories: 138; Carbohydrates: 26g; Sugar: 10g; Fiber: 6g; Fat: 4g; Saturated Fat: 1g; Protein: 2g; Sodium: 199mg

THAI GREEN VEGETABLES

SERVES 10 // PREP TIME: 20 MINUTES // COOK TIME: 3 TO 3½ HOURS

This beautiful dish is really pretty served next to a roasted chicken or pot roast. And it's fragrant and flavorful too, with the flavors of Thailand, including coconut, lime juice, chilies, lemongrass, and cilantro.

1½ pounds green beans

3 cups fresh soybeans

3 bulbs fennel, cored
  and chopped

1 jalapeño pepper, minced

1 lemongrass stalk

½ cup canned coconut milk

2 tablespoons lime juice

½ teaspoon salt

⅓ cup chopped fresh cilantro

Ⓓ Dairy-Free
Ⓖ Gluten-Free
Ⓥ Vegan

NUTRITION INFORMATION
Calories: 115; Carbohydrates; 11g;
Sugar: 4g; Fiber: 6g; Fat: 5g;
Saturated Fat: 3g; Protein: 6g;
Sodium: 154mg

1 In a 6-quart slow cooker, mix the green beans, soybeans, fennel, jalapeño pepper, lemongrass, coconut milk, lime juice, and salt. Cover and cook on low for 3 to 3½ hours, or until the vegetables are tender.

2 Remove and discard the lemongrass; sprinkle the vegetables with the cilantro and serve.

INGREDIENT TIP
Lemongrass is not edible, but it provides a lot of flavor and fragrance to recipes. To use it, rinse it well, then bend it in half. Crush it slightly with the palm of your hand and add it to the recipe. Remove and discard it when the recipe is done.

HONEYED ROOT VEGGIES

SERVES 10 // PREP TIME: 20 MINUTES // COOK TIME: 6 TO 8 HOURS

Root vegetables naturally become sweeter when they are slowly roasted, as the carbohydrates in them break down into sugar. Honey adds a sweet and floral note that makes this recipe a real treat, even though it's good for you!

6 large carrots, cut into chunks

2 onions, chopped

3 sweet potatoes, peeled and cut into chunks

2 medium rutabagas, peeled and cut into chunks

3 tablespoons honey

½ teaspoon salt

⅛ teaspoon freshly ground black pepper

In a 6-quart slow cooker, mix all of the ingredients and gently stir. Cover and cook on low for 6 to 8 hours, or until the vegetables are tender.

VARIATION TIP
Other root vegetables to use in this recipe include parsnips, russet potatoes, turnips, Yukon Gold potatoes, jicama, Jerusalem artichokes, kohlrabi, and celery root.

D Dairy-Free

G Gluten-Free

N Nut-Free

V Vegetarian

NUTRITION INFORMATION
Calories: 102; Carbohydrates: 25g;
Sugar: 14g; Fiber: 4g; Fat: 0g;
Saturated Fat: 0g; Protein: 2g;
Sodium: 177mg

BRAISED CARROT-MAPLE PURÉE

SERVES 8 // PREP TIME: 20 MINUTES // COOK TIME: 6 TO 8 HOURS

Maple syrup contains manganese, zinc, calcium, iron, potassium, and magnesium: nutrients that regular sugar doesn't. It also contains antioxidants that help prevent inflammation in the body. It's still sugar, though, so use it sparingly. It's delicious in this easy recipe.

8 large carrots, peeled and sliced

1 red onion, chopped

¼ cup canned coconut milk

2 tablespoons grated fresh ginger root

¼ cup maple syrup

½ teaspoon salt

D Dairy-Free
G Gluten-Free
V Vegan

NUTRITION INFORMATION
Calories: 80; Carbohydrates: 16g
Sugar: 11g; Fiber: 2g; Fat: 2g;
Saturated Fat: 1g; Protein: 1g;
Sodium: 203mg

1 In a 6-quart slow cooker, mix all of the ingredients. Cover and cook on low for 6 to 8 hours, or until the carrots are very tender.

2 Using a potato masher or immersion blender, puree the mixture to the desired consistency.

VARIATION TIP
You can cut the carrots into chunks instead of slices, and then don't puree the mixture. Add some dried thyme or tarragon to the carrots if you'd like.

SWEET AND SOUR RED CABBAGE

SERVES 8 // PREP TIME: 20 MINUTES // COOK TIME: 5 TO 7 HOURS

Sweet and Sour Cabbage is a classic German recipe that is perfect to serve with roasted pork or chicken. This recipe is usually made with brown sugar, but honey is substituted for a cleaner dish.

1 medium head red cabbage, cored and chopped (about 8 cups)

1 Granny Smith apple, peeled and chopped

1 red onion, chopped

3 tablespoons honey

¼ cup apple cider vinegar

½ teaspoon salt

⅛ teaspoon freshly ground black pepper

Pinch ground cloves

In a 6-quart slow cooker, mix all of the ingredients. Cover and cook on low for 5 to 7 hours, or until the cabbage is very tender.

INGREDIENT TIP
To prepare cabbage, first pull off and discard any bruised or discolored outer leaves. Cut the cabbage in half through the stem. Then cut out the core. Chop or slice the cabbage.

D Dairy-Free
G Gluten-Free
N Nut-Free
V Vegetarian

NUTRITION INFORMATION
Calories: 60; Carbohydrates: 15g; Sugar: 11g; Fiber: 3g; Fat: 0g; Saturated Fat: 0g; Protein: 1g; Sodium: 161mg

SLOW COOKER SPAGHETTI SQUASH

SERVES 8 // PREP TIME: 20 MINUTES // COOK TIME: 5 TO 7 HOURS

Spaghetti squash is a unique vegetable. When it's cooked, the flesh separates into strands that look like spaghetti pasta. Use a fork to separate the strands, then scoop them out into a bowl and top with any pasta sauce.

1 (4- to 5-pound) whole spaghetti squash, washed and dried

¼ cup water

2 tablespoons butter or coconut oil

½ teaspoon salt

⅛ teaspoon freshly ground black pepper

G Gluten-Free

V Vegetarian

NUTRITION INFORMATION
Calories: 110; Carbohydrates: 18g; Sugar: 7g; Fiber: 4g; Fat: 4g; Saturated Fat: 2g; Protein: 2g; Sodium: 214mg

1 Using a sharp knife, poke the spaghetti squash about 10 to 12 times so it doesn't explode in the slow cooker.

2 Tear off two 20-inch strips of foil. Fold each strip in half lengthwise, then in half again. In a 6-quart slow cooker, place the strips in an "X," leaving the ends draped over the outside of the appliance.

3 Place the squash onto the foil X in the slow cooker and pour in the water. Cover and cook on low for 5 to 7 hours, or until the squash is tender.

4 Carefully, using the strips, lift the squash out of the slow cooker and put it on the counter to cool for about 20 minutes.

5 Cut the squash in half crosswise. Remove the seeds with a spoon, and use a fork to separate the strands. Scoop the strands out of the squash with a large spoon.

6 Toss with the butter, salt, and pepper, and serve.

VARIATION TIP
Serve the squash with pasta sauce, Bolognese Sauce (page 32), or Beef Stroganoff (page 142). Or toss it with Parmesan cheese and serve it as a side dish.

HONEY-GLAZED TURNIPS

SERVES 8 // PREP TIME: 20 MINUTES // COOK TIME: 6 TO 8 HOURS

Turnips are a root vegetable that not many people cook anymore, although it was a staple of pioneer diets. This vegetable is very high in vitamin C, and the turnip greens are even more nutritious, with lots of manganese, calcium, and the B vitamin complex.

4 pounds turnips, peeled and sliced

1 bulk fennel, cored and chopped

2 garlic cloves, minced

¼ cup honey

¼ cup Roasted Vegetable Broth (page 30)

½ teaspoon salt

4 cups chopped turnip greens

In a 6-quart slow cooker, mix all of the ingredients. Cover and cook on low for 6 to 8 hours, or until the turnips are tender when pierced with a fork and the greens are tender too.

INGREDIENT TIP
To prepare turnips and greens, first cut the greens from the root. Peel the turnip root, then slice or cube it. Put the greens into a sink filled with cold water and swish them around to let any sand or dirt sink to the bottom. Take the greens out of the sink and dry them, then chop.

D Dairy-Free

G Gluten-Free

N Nut-Free

V Vegetarian

NUTRITION INFORMATION
Calories: 86; Carbohydrates: 20g; Sugar: 13g; Fiber: 5g; Fat: 0g; Saturated Fat: 0g; Protein: 3g; Sodium: 232mg

ITALIAN ROASTED BEETS

SERVES 8 // PREP TIME: 20 MINUTES // COOK TIME: 5 TO 7 HOURS

Beets have quite an intense flavor, in addition to their beautiful ruby red color. Adding Italian ingredients to beets changes the character of the dish. Serve this recipe with some grilled fish or pork chops.

10 medium beets, peeled and sliced

4 large tomatoes, seeded and chopped

2 onions, chopped

4 garlic cloves, minced

2 tablespoons olive oil

1 teaspoon dried basil leaves

1 teaspoon dried oregano leaves

½ teaspoon salt

1 In a 6-quart slow cooker, mix the beets, tomatoes, onions, and garlic. Drizzle with the olive oil and add the dried herbs and salt; toss to mix.

2 Cover and cook on low for 5 to 7 hours, or until the beets are tender.

VARIATION TIP
Beets and tomatoes go together very well, but you can omit the tomatoes in this recipe if you'd like. Instead, add another onion or try using cherry or grape tomatoes.

D Dairy-Free
G Gluten-Free
N Nut-Free
V Vegan

NUTRITION INFORMATION
Calories: 100; Carbohydrates: 16g;
Sugar: 10g; Fiber: 4g; Fat: 4g;
Saturated Fat: 0g; Protein: 3g;
Sodium: 215mg

EGGPLANT PARMESAN

SERVES 8 // PREP TIME: 20 MINUTES // COOK TIME: 8 TO 9 HOURS

Eggplant Parmesan is usually made by heavily salting eggplant slices, then dipping the pieces in bread crumbs, and frying them. It's delicious, but it certainly isn't a healthy or clean recipe! In this recipe, the eggplant is cooked in tomato sauce, then topped with chopped nuts to mimic the bread crumbs.

5 large eggplant, peeled and sliced ½-inch thick

2 onions, chopped

6 garlic cloves, minced

2 (8-ounce) BPA-free cans low-sodium tomato sauce

2 tablespoons olive oil

1 teaspoon dried Italian seasoning

½ cup grated Parmesan cheese

½ cup chopped toasted almonds

G Gluten-Free

V Vegetarian

NUTRITION INFORMATION
Calories: 206; Carbohydrates: 28g; Sugar: 14g; Fiber: 11g; Fat: 8g; Saturated Fat: 3g; Protein: 10g; Sodium: 283mg

1 In a 6-quart slow cooker, layer the eggplant slices with the onions and garlic.

2 In a medium bowl, mix the tomato sauce, olive oil, and Italian seasoning. Pour the tomato sauce mixture into the slow cooker.

3 Cover and cook on low for 8 to 9 hours, or until the eggplant is tender.

4 In a small bowl, mix the Parmesan cheese and almonds. Sprinkle over the eggplant mixture and serve.

VARIATION TIP
You can use other types of cheese in this rich Italian recipe, such as shredded provolone or mozzarella. Or you can omit it entirely for a vegan dish.

CRANBERRY-WALNUT GREEN BEANS

SERVES 8 // PREP TIME: 20 MINUTES // COOK TIME: 5 TO 7 HOURS

Cranberries and walnuts add color, flavor, and nutrition to plain old green beans. This is a great side dish to serve for a holiday meal.

2 pounds fresh green beans

1 onion, chopped

1 cup dried cranberries (see tip on page 68)

⅓ cup orange juice

½ teaspoon salt

⅛ teaspoon freshly ground black pepper

1 cup coarsely chopped toasted walnuts

1 In a 6-quart slow cooker, mix the green beans, onion, cranberries, orange juice, salt, and pepper. Cover and cook on low for 5 to 7 hours, or until the green beans are tender.

2 Add the walnuts and serve.

INGREDIENT TIP
To toast nuts, spread them on a cookie sheet and bake in a 375°F oven for about 5 to 10 minutes. You'll know when the nuts are done when they are fragrant. Remove and let cool before you chop them, or the nuts will be greasy.

D Dairy-Free

G Gluten-Free

V Vegan

NUTRITION INFORMATION
Calories: 100; Carbohydrates: 18g; Sugar: 11g; Fiber: 3g; Fat: 3g; Saturated Fat: 0g; Protein: 2g; Sodium: 151mg

TEX-MEX CORN AND TOMATOES

SERVES 8 // PREP TIME: 20 MINUTES // COOK TIME: 5 TO 6 HOURS

This easy and colorful recipe can be served as a side dish when you make tacos, or it is great with grilled steak or roasted chicken. Make it as spicy or mild as you like by varying the amounts of jalapeños you add.

5 cups frozen corn

4 large tomatoes, seeded and chopped

2 onions, chopped

4 garlic cloves, minced

2 jalapeño peppers, minced

1 tablespoon chili powder

½ teaspoon salt

⅛ teaspoon cayenne pepper

In a 6-quart slow cooker, mix all the ingredients. Cover and cook on low for 5 to 6 hours, or until the onions are tender.

INGREDIENT TIP
If you prefer, you can use fresh corn kernels in place of the frozen ones. To cut kernels from a corncob, hold the cob upright in the hole of a bundt pan. Cut down with a sharp knife to remove the kernels. They will fall right into the bundt pan instead of scattering around the kitchen.

Ⓓ Dairy-Free

Ⓖ Gluten-Free

Ⓝ Nut-Free

Ⓥ Vegan

NUTRITION INFORMATION
Calories: 124; Carbohydrates: 29g; Sugar: 14g; Fiber: 5g; Fat: 1g; Saturated Fat: 0g; Protein: 4g; Sodium: 167mg

BALSAMIC-GLAZED VEGGIES OVER COUSCOUS

SERVES 10 // PREP TIME: 20 MINUTES // COOK TIME: 7 TO 9 HOURS

Balsamic vinegar has a naturally sweet flavor that complements the sweetness of these vegetables. You can use any kind of root vegetable you'd like in this easy recipe. It's the perfect side dish to a roasted chicken or meatloaf.

2 sweet potatoes, peeled and cubed

10 garlic cloves, peeled and sliced

4 large carrots, peeled and cut into chunks

2 zucchinis, cut into chunks

2 (10-ounce) BPA-free cans no-salt-added artichoke hearts in water, drained

¼ cup balsamic vinegar

2 tablespoons honey

1 teaspoon dried marjoram leaves

5 cups whole-wheat couscous, cooked according to package directions

D Dairy-Free

N Nut-Free

V Vegetarian

1 In a 6-quart slow cooker, mix the sweet potatoes, garlic, carrots, zucchinis, artichoke hearts, vinegar, honey, and marjoram leaves. Cover and cook on low for 7 to 9 hours, or until the vegetables are tender.

2 Serve over the hot cooked couscous.

INGREDIENT TIP
Balsamic vinegar is made of grape must (whole pressed grapes) that is fermented and then aged in wooden casks. It can be very expensive, especially if it is aged for decades. But you can buy relatively good balsamic vinegar in any grocery store.

NUTRITION INFORMATION
Calories: 173; Carbohydrates: 36g; Sugar: 9g; Fiber: 5g; Fat: 1g; Saturated Fat: 0g; Protein: 5g; Sodium: 53mg

BRAISED CABBAGE AND ONIONS

SERVES 8 // PREP TIME: 20 MINUTES // COOK TIME: 6 TO 7 HOURS

Cabbage is so good for you, and it's so inexpensive. It's braised in vegetable broth and vinegar in this easy recipe, which is delicious to serve with pork chops or grilled chicken.

1 large head green cabbage, cored and chopped

3 onions, chopped

6 garlic cloves, minced

½ cup Roasted Vegetable Broth (page 30)

2 tablespoons apple cider vinegar

2 tablespoons honey

1 tablespoons olive oil

½ teaspoon salt

G Gluten-Free

N Nut-Free

V Vegetarian

NUTRITION INFORMATION
Calories: 75; Carbohydrates: 14g;
Sugar: 10g; Fiber: 3g; Fat: 2g;
Saturated Fat: 0g; Protein: 2g;
Sodium: 171mg

In a 6-quart slow cooker, mix all of the ingredients. Cover and cook on low for 6 to 7 hours, or until the cabbage and onions are tender.

INGREDIENT TIP
Cabbage is a cruciferous vegetable, which means it contains antioxidants that can help protect against cancer. Both red and green cabbage are high in vitamins K and C.

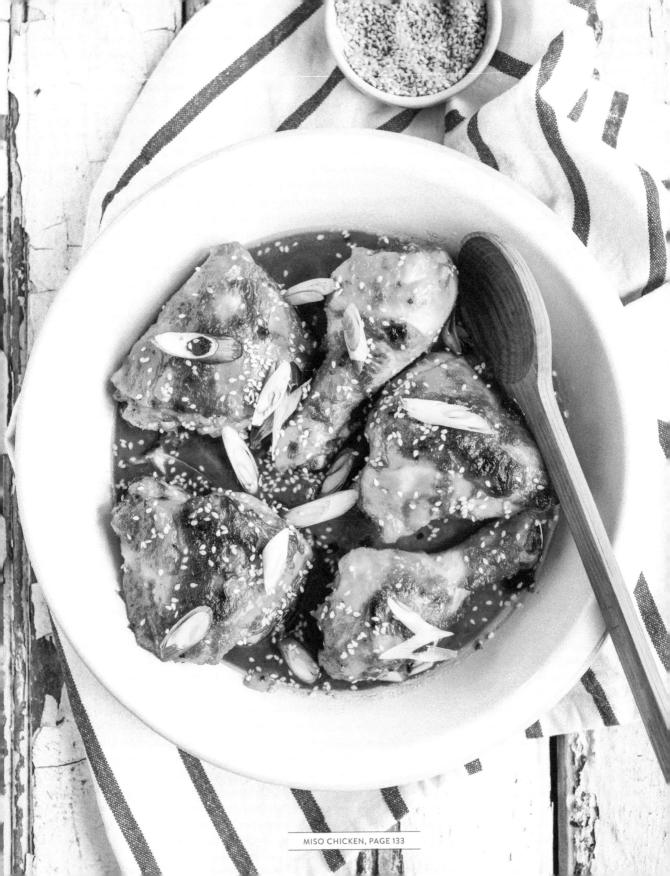

MISO CHICKEN, PAGE 133

CHAPTER EIGHT

SEAFOOD AND POULTRY

SALMON WITH ROOT VEGETABLES

SERVES 6 // PREP TIME: 20 MINUTES // COOK TIME: 7 ½ TO 9 ½ HOURS

Salmon cooks beautifully in the slow cooker, but it takes only about 30 minutes for a fillet to cook. So we'll cook root vegetables for hours until they are tender and sweet, then add the salmon just before you're ready to eat.

4 large carrots, sliced

2 sweet potatoes, peeled and cubed

4 Yukon Gold potatoes, cubed

2 onions, chopped

3 garlic cloves, minced

⅓ cup Roasted Vegetable Broth (page 30) or Fish Stock (page 28)

1 teaspoon dried thyme leaves

½ teaspoon salt

6 (5-ounce) salmon fillets

⅓ cup grated Parmesan cheese

1 In a 6-quart slow cooker, mix carrots, sweet potatoes, Yukon Gold potatoes, onions, garlic, vegetable broth, thyme, and salt. Cover and cook on low for 7 to 9 hours, or until the vegetables are tender.

2 Add the salmon fillets and sprinkle each with some of the cheese. Cover and cook on low for 30 to 40 minutes, or until the salmon flakes when tested with a fork.

SUBSTITUTION TIP
You can cook other types of fish fillets in this recipe too. But most white fish fillets, such as red snapper or halibut, will take only about 20 minutes to cook in the slow cooker.

Ⓖ Gluten-Free

Ⓝ Nut-Free

NUTRITION INFORMATION
Calories: 491; Carbohydrates: 38g;
Sugar: 8g; Fiber: 5g; Fat: 19g;
Saturated Fat: 4g; Protein: 42g;
Sodium: 560mg

WHITE FISH RISOTTO

SERVES 6 // PREP TIME: 20 MINUTES // COOK TIME: 3½ TO 4 HOURS 45 MINUTES

You can use vegetable broth or fish stock for the liquid in this wonderful and rich recipe. Make your own fish stock, using the recipe on page 28, or buy the fish stock from a fishmonger.

8-ounces cremini mushrooms, sliced

2 onions, chopped

5 garlic cloves, minced

2 cups short-grain brown rice

1 teaspoon dried thyme leaves

6 cups Roasted Vegetable Broth (page 30) or Fish Stock (page 28)

6 (5-ounce) tilapia fillets

2 cups baby spinach leaves

2 tablespoons unsalted butter

½ cup grated Parmesan cheese

G Gluten-Free

N Nut-Free

NUTRITION INFORMATION
Calories: 469; Carbohydrate: 61g; Sugar: 2g; Fiber: 5g; Fat: 12g; Saturated Fat: 5g; Protein: 34g; Sodium: 346mg

1 In a 6-quart slow cooker, mix the mushrooms, onions, garlic, rice, thyme, and vegetable broth. Cover and cook on low for 3 to 4 hours, or until the rice is tender.

2 Put the fish on top of the rice. Cover and cook for 25 to 35 minutes longer, or until the fish flakes when tested with a fork.

3 Gently stir the fish into the risotto. Add the baby spinach leaves.

4 Stir in the butter and cheese. Cover and let cook on low for 10 minutes, then serve.

INGREDIENT TIP
Fish is good for you, but certain species should be avoided because of mercury concerns. Don't eat imported swordfish, tilefish, marlin, or tuna steaks. Red snapper is fine to eat once a week, and you can eat cod, pollock, trout, and tilapia 2 to 3 times a week.

CARROT MÉLANGE WITH POACHED FISH

SERVES 6 // PREP TIME: 20 MINUTES // COOK TIME: 7½ TO 9½ HOURS

Carrots come in many different colors, and you can find them in most large supermarkets and at farmers' markets. Purple, red, white, and yellow carrots make this recipe so pretty and colorful. And it tastes great too!

4 large orange carrots, peeled and sliced

3 yellow carrots, peeled and sliced

3 purple carrots, peeled and sliced

2 onions, chopped

4 garlic cloves, minced

½ cup Roasted Vegetable Broth (page 30) or Fish Stock (page 28)

1 teaspoon dried marjoram leaves

1 bay leaf

½ teaspoon salt

6 (5-ounce) trout fillets

1 In a 6-quart slow cooker, mix the carrots, onions, garlic, vegetable broth, marjoram, bay leaf, and salt. Cover and cook on low for 7 to 9 hours, or until the carrots are tender.

2 Remove and discard the bay leaf.

3 Add the trout fillets to the slow cooker. Cover and cook on low for 20 to 30 minutes, or until the fish flakes when tested with a fork.

SUBSTITUTION TIP
Use other root vegetables in place of the more exotic colored carrots. Kohlrabi, jicama, or celery root would be a nice change of pace.

Ⓓ Dairy-Free
Ⓖ Gluten-Free
Ⓝ Nut-Free

NUTRITION INFORMATION
Calories: 263; Carbohydrates: 19g; Sugar: 9g; Fiber: 5g; Fat: 9g; Saturated Fat: 3g; Protein: 28g; Sodium: 357mg

SALMON AND BARLEY BAKE

SERVES 6 // PREP TIME: 20 MINUTES // COOK TIME: 7 ½ TO 8 ½ HOURS

Fennel is a root vegetable that tastes like licorice. It is complemented by the tarragon in this recipe, which also has a faint licorice flavor.

2 cups hulled barley, rinsed

2 fennel bulbs, cored
and chopped

2 red bell peppers, stemmed,
seeded, and chopped

4 garlic cloves, minced

1 (8-ounce) package cremini
mushrooms, sliced

5 cups Roasted Vegetable
Broth (page 30)

1 teaspoon dried
tarragon leaves

⅛ teaspoon freshly ground
black pepper

6 (5-ounce) salmon fillets

⅓ cup grated
Parmesan cheese

1 In a 6-quart slow cooker, mix the barley, fennel, bell peppers, garlic, mushrooms, vegetable broth, tarragon, and pepper. Cover and cook on low for 7 to 8 hours, or until the barley has absorbed most of the liquid and is tender, and the vegetables are tender too.

2 Place the salmon fillets on top of the barley mixture. Cover and cook on low for 20 to 40 minutes longer, or until the salmon flakes when tested with a fork.

3 Stir in the Parmesan cheese, breaking up the salmon, and serve.

SUBSTITUTION TIP
If you don't like the taste of licorice, substitute 2 chopped leeks for the fennel, and use dried basil or thyme leaves in place of the tarragon.

Ⓝ Nut-Free

NUTRITION INFORMATION
Calories: 609; Carbohydrates: 55g;
Sugar: 4g; Fiber: 13g; Fat: 20g;
Saturated Fat: 4g; Protein: 49g;
Sodium: 441mg

SALMON RATATOUILLE

SERVES 8 // PREP TIME: 20 MINUTES // COOK TIME: 6½ TO 7½ HOURS

Ratatouille is a classic vegetarian dish. Add some salmon to turn it into a main dish with extra flavor and nutrition. You could add other types of fish instead; tilapia or halibut fillets would be delicious.

2 eggplant, peeled and chopped

5 large tomatoes, seeded and chopped

2 cups sliced button mushrooms

2 onions, chopped

2 red bell peppers, stemmed, seeded, and chopped

5 garlic cloves, minced

2 tablespoons olive oil

1 teaspoon dried herbes de Provence

2 pounds salmon fillets

1 In a 6-quart slow cooker, mix the eggplant, tomatoes, mushrooms, onions, bell peppers, garlic, olive oil, and herbes de Provence. Cover and cook on low for 6 to 7 hours, or until the vegetables are tender.

2 Add the salmon to the slow cooker. Cover and cook on low for 30 to 40 minutes, or until the salmon flakes when tested with a fork.

3 Gently stir the salmon into the vegetables and serve.

RECIPE TIP
Most recipes call for salting eggplant to get rid of bitter flavors and to remove some of the liquid. But eggplant grown today is bred to not be so bitter, so you can skip that step.

D Dairy-Free

G Gluten-Free

N Nut-Free

NUTRITION INFORMATION
Calories: 342; Carbohydrates: 18g; Sugar: 10g; Fiber: 7g; Fat: 16g; Saturated Fat: 2g; Protein: 32g; Sodium: 218mg

JERK CHICKEN

SERVES 8 // PREP TIME: 20 MINUTES // COOK TIME: 7 TO 9 HOURS

This spicy and easy recipe deeply infuses chicken with a rich and hot flavor. Serve it with brown rice and some sautéed or slow cooked vegetables to soak up the sauce.

10 (4-ounce) boneless, skinless chicken thighs

2 tablespoons honey

3 tablespoons grated fresh ginger root

1 teaspoon ground red chili

1 tablespoon chili powder

½ teaspoon ground cloves

¼ teaspoon ground allspice

3 onions, chopped

6 garlic cloves, minced

½ cup freshly squeezed orange juice

Ⓓ Dairy-Free
Ⓖ Gluten-Free
Ⓝ Nut-Free

NUTRITION INFORMATION
Calories: 184; Carbohydrates: 11g; Sugar: 7g; Fiber: 1g; Fat: 3g; Saturated Fat: 1g; Protein: 30g; Sodium: 316mg

1 Cut slashes across the chicken thighs so the flavorings can permeate.

2 In a small bowl, mix the honey, ginger root, ground chili, chili powder, cloves, and allspice. Rub this mixture into the chicken. Let the chicken stand while you prepare the vegetables.

3 In the bottom of a 6-quart slow cooker, place the onions and garlic. Top with the chicken. Pour the orange juice over all. Cover and cook on low for 7 to 9 hours, or until a food thermometer registers 165°F.

INGREDIENT TIP
"Jerk" is a type of cooking and a type of seasoning. The cooking style is from Jamaica, and it means the meat is marinated in a spice mixture. Jerk seasoning is a combination of chili peppers, cloves, allspice, ginger, garlic, and cinnamon.

VEGETABLE SHRIMP SCAMPI

SERVES 8 // PREP TIME: 20 MINUTES // COOK TIME: 5½ TO 7½ HOURS

Shrimp is not something you usually associate with cooking in the slow cooker. But with a few tweaks, shrimp cooks very well in this appliance. This easy recipe is a treat and something you can serve to company.

1 pound cremini mushrooms, sliced

2 onions, chopped

2 leeks, chopped

8 garlic cloves, minced

1 cup Fish Stock (page 28)

¼ cup freshly squeezed lemon juice

1 teaspoon dried basil leaves

2 pounds raw shrimp, shelled and deveined

2 tablespoons butter

Ⓖ Gluten-Free

Ⓝ Nut-Free

NUTRITION INFORMATION
Calories: 158; Carbohydrates: 10g; Sugar: 3g; Fiber: 2g; Fat: 4g; Saturated Fat: 2g; Protein: 22g; Sodium: 275mg

1 In a 6-quart slow cooker, mix the mushrooms, onions, leeks, garlic, fish stock, lemon juice, and basil. Cover and cook on low for 5 to 7 hours, or until the vegetables are tender.

2 Stir in the shrimp. Cover and cook on high for 30 to 40 minutes, or until the shrimp curl and turn pink.

3 Stir in the butter; cover and let stand for 10 minutes, then serve.

INGREDIENT TIP
When you buy shrimp, look for the ones labeled Aquaculture Stewardship Council or Responsibly Farmed. Shrimp can be problematic if it is raised on a farm overseas, containing chemicals and bacteria. Buy responsibly caught US wild shrimp if you can.

JAMBALAYA

SERVES 8 // PREP TIME: 20 MINUTES // COOK TIME: 7½ TO 9½ HOURS

Jambalaya is a Cajun recipe that is a combination of chicken, sausage, shrimp, and vegetables. It's usually very spicy, although you can vary the level of heat to suit your tastes. This delicious recipe is good for you too, since we omit the sausage, which is high in fat and sodium.

10 (4-ounce) boneless, skinless chicken thighs, cut into 2-inch pieces

2 onions, chopped

6 garlic cloves, minced

2 jalapeño peppers, minced

2 green bell peppers, stemmed, seeded, and chopped

5 celery stalks, sliced

2 cups Chicken Stock (page 26)

1 tablespoon Cajun seasoning

¼ teaspoon cayenne pepper

1½ pounds raw shrimp, shelled and deveined

1 In a 6-quart slow cooker, mix the chicken, onions, garlic, jalapeños, bell peppers, celery, chicken stock, Cajun seasoning, and cayenne. Cover and cook on low for 7 to 9 hours, or until the chicken registers 165°F on a food thermometer.

2 Stir in the shrimp. Cover and cook for another 30 to 40 minutes, or until the shrimp curl and turn pink.

VARIATION TIP
Serve this recipe with some cooked brown rice. The traditional way to serve it is to put a scoop of brown rice on top of the jambalaya in the bowl. This way the rice doesn't get soggy and you can scoop some up with every spoonful.

D Dairy-Free
G Gluten-Free
N Nut-Free

NUTRITION INFORMATION
Calories: 417; Carbohydrates: 27g;
Sugar: 3g; Fiber: 3g; Fat: 20g;
Saturated Fat: 5g; Protein: 34g;
Sodium: 385mg

ROASTED CHICKEN WITH SQUASH

SERVES 8 // PREP TIME: 20 MINUTES // COOK TIME: 6 TO 8 HOURS

Chicken and squash make a great combination, especially when cooked in the slow cooker, because the chicken stays moist and tender.

1 (3-pound) butternut squash, peeled, seeded, and cut into 1-inch pieces

2 (1-pound) acorn squash, peeled, seeded, and cut into 1-inch pieces

2 fennel bulbs, cored and sliced

1 (8-ounce) package cremini mushrooms, sliced

8 (6-ounce) bone-in, skinless chicken breasts

3 sprigs fresh thyme

1 bay leaf

1 cup Chicken Stock (page 26)

½ cup canned coconut milk

2 tablespoons lemon juice

D Dairy-Free
G Gluten-Free

NUTRITION INFORMATION
Calories: 330; Carbohydrates: 21g; Sugar: 3g; Fiber: 4g; Fat: 8g; Saturated Fat: 3g; Protein: 43g; Sodium: 67mg

1 In a 6-quart slow cooker, mix the butternut squash, acorn squash, fennel, mushrooms, chicken, thyme, bay leaf, chicken stock, and coconut milk. Cover and cook on low for 6 to 8 hours, or until the chicken registers 165°F on a food thermometer.

2 Remove and discard the thyme sprigs and bay leaf. Stir in the lemon juice and serve.

VARIATION TIP
You can make this recipe with bone-in, skinless chicken thighs too. The cooking time may increase slightly. Or you can remove the chicken from the slow cooker when it's done, remove the bones, and cut the chicken into large chunks, then return it to the slow cooker and serve.

SHRIMP AND GRITS

SERVES 8 // PREP TIME: 20 MINUTES // COOK TIME: 5½ TO 7½ HOURS

This classic Southern recipe is a great choice for the slow cooker. Grits are ground cornmeal and considered a whole grain. The grits cook in chicken broth and seasonings for hours; then the shrimp is added and cooked until tender.

2½ cups stone-ground grits

2 onions, chopped

5 garlic cloves, minced

4 large tomatoes, seeded and chopped

2 green bell peppers, stemmed, seeded, and chopped

8 cups Chicken Stock (page 26) or Roasted Vegetable Broth (page 30)

1 bay leaf

1 teaspoon Old Bay® Seasoning

2 pounds raw shrimp, peeled and deveined

1½ cups shredded Cheddar cheese

Ⓖ Gluten-Free

Ⓝ Nut-Free

NUTRITION INFORMATION
Calories: 415; Carbohydrates: 51g;
Sugar: 5g; Fiber: 5g; Fat: 10g;
Saturated Fat: 4g; Protein: 33g;
Sodium: 415mg

1 In a 6-quart slow cooker, mix the grits, onions, garlic, tomatoes, bell peppers, chicken stock, bay leaf, and seasoning. Cover and cook on low for 5 to 7 hours, or until the grits are tender and most of the liquid is absorbed.

2 Add the shrimp and stir. Cover and cook on low for 30 to 40 minutes longer, or until the shrimp curl and turn pink.

3 Stir in the cheese and serve.

INGREDIENT TIP
Old Bay® Seasoning is a classic spice mix used with sea-food. It is made of celery salt, red pepper, paprika, ground bay leaf, cloves, allspice, and lots of pepper. You can make your own if you can't find it at the store.

THAI CHICKEN AND GREENS

SERVES 8 // PREP TIME: 20 MINUTES // COOK TIME: 6 TO 8 HOURS

Leafy greens are so good for you, and they are delicious when cooked in the slow cooker with chicken and Thai seasonings.

2 (16-ounce) packages prepared collard greens

2 cups chopped kale

2 onions, chopped

6 garlic cloves, minced

2 red chili peppers, minced

1 lemongrass stalk

10 (4-ounce) boneless, skinless chicken thighs

1 cup Chicken Stock (page 26)

1 cup canned coconut milk

3 tablespoons freshly squeezed lime juice

D Dairy-Free
G Gluten-Free

NUTRITION INFORMATION
Calories: 338; Carbohydrates:15g;
Sugar: 3g; Fiber: 7g; Fat: 17g;
Saturated Fat: 9g; Protein: 33g;
Sodium: 173mg

1 In a 6-quart slow cooker, mix the greens and kale and top with the onions, garlic, chili peppers, lemongrass, and chicken. Pour the chicken stock and coconut milk over all.

2 Cover and cook on low for 6 to 8 hours, or until the chicken registers 165°F on a food thermometer and the greens are tender.

3 Remove and discard the lemongrass. Stir in the lime juice and serve.

INGREDIENT TIP
You can buy prewashed collard greens in many grocery stores now, which saves a lot of preparation time. If you can't find them, put the greens into a sink of cold water. Swish the greens around to remove any sand. Then pull the leaves off the stems (discard the stems) and use.

MISO CHICKEN

SERVES 8 // PREP TIME: 20 MINUTES // COOK TIME: 7 TO 8 HOURS

This recipe has so much flavor. Miso paste is made from fermented soybeans. This Asian ingredient is delicious cooked with tender chicken in this simple recipe. You could use skinless chicken breasts if you'd like; in that case, the cooking time will be reduced by about an hour.

1 onion, chopped

3 garlic cloves, minced

2 tablespoons grated fresh ginger root

2 pounds skinless chicken drumsticks

2 pounds skinless chicken thighs

2 cups Chicken Stock (page 26), divided

2 tablespoons honey

2 tablespoons miso paste

2 tablespoons toasted sesame seeds

4 scallions, cut on the bias

D Dairy-Free

G Gluten-Free

N Nut-Free

1 In a 6-quart slow cooker, mix the onion, garlic, and ginger root. Top with the chicken drumsticks and thighs.

2 In a medium bowl, mix ½ cup of the chicken stock with the honey and miso paste and whisk to blend. Add the remaining 1½ cups of the chicken stock and mix until well blended, then pour this mixture into the slow cooker.

3 Cover and cook on low for 7 to 8 hours, or until the chicken registers 165°F on a food thermometer.

4 Sprinkle with the sesame seeds and scallions and serve.

INGREDIENT TIP
Miso paste can be high in sodium. But research has shown the sodium in this particular ingredient does not adversely affect your health. Miso has a very intense taste. The darker the miso, the more flavorful it is.

NUTRITION INFORMATION
Calories: 405; Carbohydrates: 10g; Sugar: 7g; Fiber: 1g; Fat: 19g; Saturated Fat: 4g; Protein: 48g; Sodium: 529mg

CHICKEN WITH ARTICHOKES

SERVES 8 // PREP TIME: 20 MINUTES // COOK TIME: 4 TO 6 HOURS

Artichokes seem like an exotic food, and I always wonder who decided to eat the first one. But you can buy frozen and canned artichoke hearts that are already prepared so you don't have to do all the work of removing the leaves and the choke to get to its center. This colorful dish is rich and delicious.

2 leeks, chopped

3 garlic cloves, minced

2 (14-ounce) BPA-free cans
no-salt-added artichoke
hearts, drained

2 red bell peppers, stemmed,
seeded, and chopped

8 (6-ounce) boneless,
skinless chicken breasts

1 cup Chicken Stock
(page 26)

2 tablespoons lemon juice

1 teaspoon dried basil leaves

½ cup chopped
flat-leaf parsley

1 In a 6-quart slow cooker, layer the leeks, garlic, artichoke hearts, bell peppers, chicken, stock, lemon juice, and basil. Cover and cook on low for 4 to 6 hours, or until the chicken registers 165°F on a food thermometer.

2 Sprinkle with the parsley and serve.

INGREDIENT TIP
Artichokes are full of fiber and are a great source of antioxidants that help protect against cancer and heart disease. And they are a great source of vitamin K, folic acid, and potassium.

Ⓓ Dairy-Free
Ⓖ Gluten-Free
Ⓝ Nut-Free

NUTRITION INFORMATION
Calories: 200; Carbohydrates: 7g;
Sugar: 2g; Fiber: 3g; Fat: 4g;
Saturated Fat: 1g; Protein: 36g;
Sodium: 372mg

CHICKEN PROVENÇAL

SERVES 8 // PREP TIME: 20 MINUTES // COOK TIME: 7 TO 9 HOURS

Food from Provence is rich, colorful, and full of flavor. Tomatoes, onions, garlic, fennel, thyme, and basil make this dish really good, and the chicken thighs stay tender and juicy when cooked in the slow cooker.

3 pounds boneless, skinless chicken thighs

3 bulbs fennel, cored and sliced

2 red bell peppers, stemmed, seeded, and chopped

2 onions, chopped

6 garlic cloves, minced

4 large tomatoes, seeded and chopped

4 sprigs fresh thyme

1 bay leaf

¼ cup sliced black Greek olives

2 tablespoons lemon juice

1　In a 6-quart slow cooker, mix all of the ingredients. Cover and cook on low for 7 to 9 hours, or until the chicken registers 165°F on a food thermometer.

2　Remove and discard the thyme stems and bay leaf and serve.

INGREDIENT TIP
Black olives are olives that have been left to ripen on the tree. They have a richer and more mellow flavor than green olives. They are high in sodium, though, so use them sparingly.

Ⓓ Dairy-Free
Ⓖ Gluten-Free
Ⓝ Nut-Free

NUTRITION INFORMATION
Calories: 302; Carbohydrates: 13g;
Sugar: 7g; Fiber: 4g; Fat: 14g;
Saturated Fat: 4g; Protein: 34g;
Sodium: 187mg

BBQ CHICKEN

SERVES 8 // PREP TIME: 20 MINUTES // COOK TIME: 5 TO 7 HOURS

Chicken cooked in a homemade barbecue sauce tastes nothing like what you get at a fast-food restaurant, or, for that matter, cooked in a purchased barbecue sauce. Serve this recipe with some coleslaw and potato salad.

2 (8-ounce) BPA-free cans no-salt-added tomato sauce

2 onions, minced

8 garlic cloves, minced

⅓ cup mustard

2 tablespoons lemon juice

3 tablespoons molasses

1 tablespoon chili powder

2 teaspoons paprika

¼ teaspoon cayenne pepper

8 (6-ounce) boneless, skinless chicken breasts

Ⓓ Dairy-Free
Ⓖ Gluten-Free
Ⓝ Nut-Free

NUTRITION INFORMATION
Calories: 231; Carbohydrates: 16g;
Sugar: 10g; Fiber: 2g; Fat: 4g;
Saturated Fat: 1g; Protein: 35g;
Sodium: 490mg

1 In a 6-quart slow cooker, mix the tomato sauce, onions, garlic, mustard, lemon juice, molasses, chili powder, paprika, and cayenne.

2 Add the chicken and use tongs to move the chicken around in the sauce to coat. Cover and cook on low for 5 to 7 hours, or until the chicken registers 165°F on a food thermometer.

VARIATION TIP
You can take the chicken out of the sauce, shred the chicken with two forks, put it back in the sauce, and serve on toasted whole-wheat buns for a nice twist.

BUTTER CHICKEN

SERVES 8 // PREP TIME: 20 MINUTES // COOK TIME: 7 ½ TO 9 ½ HOURS

Despite its name, Butter Chicken doesn't contain any butter! This Indian dish is called Butter Chicken because the chicken becomes as soft as butter when it's cooked with these ingredients. Yogurt, curry powder, and lemon juice coat and flavor the chicken as it cooks.

½ cup plain Greek yogurt

⅓ cup lemon juice

5 teaspoons curry powder

2 tablespoons grated fresh ginger root

10 (4-ounce) boneless, skinless chicken thighs

4 large tomatoes, seeded and chopped

2 onions, chopped

8 garlic cloves, sliced

⅔ cup canned coconut milk

3 tablespoons cornstarch

D Dairy-Free

G Gluten-Free

NUTRITION INFORMATION
Calories: 295; Carbohydrates: 12g;
Sugar: 5g; Fiber: 2g; Fat: 15g;
Saturated Fat: 7g; Protein: 30g;
Sodium: 124mg

1   In a medium bowl, mix the yogurt, lemon juice, curry powder, and ginger root. Add the chicken and stir to coat; let stand for 15 minutes while you prepare the other ingredients.

2   In a 6-quart slow cooker, mix the tomatoes, onions, and garlic.

3   Add the chicken-yogurt mixture to the slow cooker. Cover and cook on low for 7 to 9 hours, or until the chicken registers 165°F on a food thermometer.

4   In a small bowl, mix the coconut milk and cornstarch. Stir into the slow cooker.

5   Cover and cook on low for another 15 to 20 minutes, or until the sauce has thickened.

SUBSTITUTION TIP
You can use 8 boneless, skinless chicken breasts in place of the thighs in this recipe if you'd like. The cooking time should be reduced to 5 to 7 hours on low.

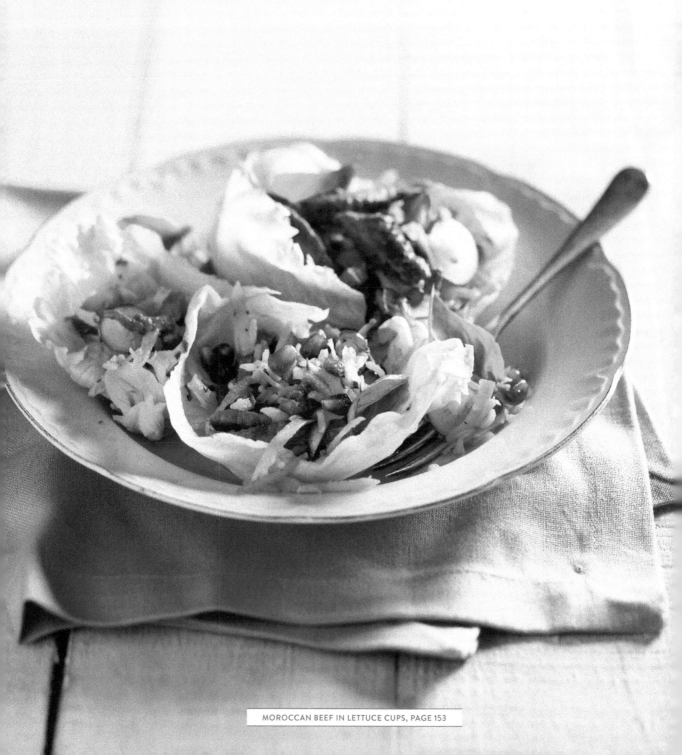

MOROCCAN BEEF IN LETTUCE CUPS, PAGE 153

CHAPTER NINE

PORK AND BEEF

GINGERED PORK CHOPS

SERVES 8 // PREP TIME: 20 MINUTES // COOK TIME: 6 TO 8 HOURS

Pork chops cook beautifully in the slow cooker. This cut can be tough and dry if fried or baked, but the slow cooker makes the meat very tender and juicy. This flavorful recipe is very easy to make.

2 onions, chopped

3 garlic cloves, minced

4 large carrots, peeled and cut into chunks

8 (5-ounce) pork chops

3 tablespoons grated fresh ginger root

3 tablespoons honey

½ cup Chicken Stock (page 26)

½ teaspoon ground ginger

½ teaspoon salt

⅛ teaspoon freshly ground black pepper

1 In a 6-quart slow cooker, mix the onions, garlic, and carrots. Top with the pork chops.

2 In a small bowl, mix the ginger root, honey, stock, ginger, salt, and pepper. Pour into the slow cooker.

3 Cover and cook on low for 6 to 8 hours, or until the pork is very tender.

RECIPE TIP
You can brown the pork chops in a skillet over medium heat before you add them to the slow cooker if you'd like. This adds to the appearance and enhances the flavor of the pork, but this step isn't necessary for the recipe to work.

D Dairy-Free

G Gluten-Free

N Nut-Free

NUTRITION INFORMATION
Calories: 241; Carbohydrates: 15g; Sugar: 11g; Fiber: 2g; Fat: 6g; Saturated Fat: 2g; Protein: 32g; Sodium: 267mg

SAVORY POT ROAST

SERVES 8 // PREP TIME: 20 MINUTES // COOK TIME: 8 TO 10 HOURS

Pot roast is one of the most comforting recipes around, if you are not a vegetarian. An inexpensive cut of beef becomes meltingly tender when cooked in the slow cooker.

8 Yukon Gold potatoes, cut into chunks

4 large carrots, peeled and cut into chunks

2 onions, chopped

1 leek, sliced

8 garlic cloves, sliced

1 (3-pound) grass-fed chuck shoulder roast or tri-tip roast

1 teaspoon dried marjoram

½ teaspoon salt

¼ teaspoon freshly ground black pepper

1 cup Beef Stock (page 27)

D Dairy-Free
G Gluten-Free
N Nut-Free

NUTRITION INFORMATION
Calories: 567; Carbohydrates: 36g;
Sugar: 5g; Fiber: 4g; Fat: 31g;
Saturated Fat: 12g; Protein: 37g;
Sodium: 301mg

1 In a 6-quart slow cooker, mix the potatoes, carrots, onions, leek, and garlic.

2 Place the beef on top of the vegetables and sprinkle with the marjoram, salt, and pepper.

3 Pour the beef stock into the slow cooker.

4 Cover and cook on low for 8 to 10 hours, or until the beef is very tender. Serve the beef with the vegetables.

INGREDIENT TIP
Try to find grass-fed beef when you are following the eating clean plan. This type of beef is usually hormone-free, and the animals are raised without antibiotics. It's also better for the environment, since the farmers don't have to import grain to feed the cattle.

CLEAN BEEF STROGANOFF

SERVES 8 // PREP TIME: 20 MINUTES // COOK TIME: 7½ TO 9½ HOURS

Beef Stroganoff is a classic dish made of beef simmered with vegetables in a stock. The sauce is thickened with sour cream, then the whole thing is served over noodles. This clean version is better than the original.

2 onions, chopped

2 cups sliced cremini mushrooms

5 large carrots, sliced

8 garlic cloves, sliced

2½ pounds grass-fed chuck shoulder roast, trimmed of fat and cut in 2-inch cubes

2 cups Beef Stock (page 27)

3 tablespoons mustard

1 bay leaf

1 teaspoon dried marjoram

1½ cups sour cream

3 tablespoons cornstarch

G Gluten-Free

N Nut-Free

NUTRITION INFORMATION
Calories: 503; Carbohydrates: 15g; Sugar: 6g; Fiber: 2g; Fat: 33g; Saturated Fat: 16g; Protein: 32g; Sodium: 246mg

1 In a 6-quart slow cooker, mix the onions, mushrooms, carrots, garlic, and beef.

2 In a medium bowl, mix the beef stock and mustard. Add the bay leaf and marjoram and pour into the slow cooker.

3 Cover and cook on low for 7 to 9 hours, or until the beef is very tender.

4 In a medium bowl, mix the sour cream and cornstarch. Add 1 cup of the liquid from the slow cooker and whisk until well blended.

5 Add the sour cream mixture to the slow cooker. Cover and cook on low for 20 to 30 minutes, or until the liquid has thickened. Discard the bay leaf and serve.

VARIATION TIP
You can serve this over hot cooked whole-wheat noodles, or serve it over mashed cauliflower or potatoes. Beef Stroganoff is also good served over polenta.

BEEF AND BEAN BURRITO CASSEROLE

SERVES 8 // PREP TIME: 20 MINUTES // COOK TIME: 5 TO 7 HOURS

A burrito is a Tex-Mex dish made of a richly seasoned filling rolled up in a tortilla. In this clean version, corn tortillas are layered with a mixture of beef, vegetables, and beans.

1½ pounds grass-fed lean ground beef

2 onions, chopped

4 garlic cloves, minced

2 jalapeño peppers, minced

1 (16-ounce) BPA-free can no-salt-added vegetarian refried beans

1 (15-ounce) BPA-free can no-salt-added black beans, drained and rinsed

1 tablespoon chili powder

1 teaspoon dried oregano

8 corn tortillas

2 cups shredded white Cheddar cheese

Ⓖ Gluten-Free

Ⓝ Nut-Free

NUTRITION INFORMATION
Calories: 553; Carbohydrates: 34g; Sugar: 5g; Fiber: 8g; Fat: 28g; Saturated Fat: 13g; Protein: 39g; Sodium: 517mg

1 In a large saucepan, cook the beef, onions, and garlic over medium-high heat for 8 to 10 minutes, stirring to break up the meat. Drain well.

2 Add the jalapeño peppers, refried beans, black beans, chili powder, and oregano to the beef mixture.

3 In a 6-quart slow cooker, layer the beef mixture with the tortillas and shredded cheese.

4 Cover and cook on low for 5 to 7 hours, or until the tortillas have softened.

INGREDIENT TIP
When you buy canned vegetarian refried beans, look for a BPA-free can. Then read the ingredient list. It should contain beans, some type of oil, and salt. That's it. This recipe calls for vegetarian beans because the nonvegetarian variety is usually made with lard.

HERBED PORK LOIN WITH FRUIT

SERVES 8 // PREP TIME: 20 MINUTES // COOK TIME: 7 TO 9 HOURS

Meat with fruit is a great combination that is not only delicious, but also healthy. The sweet taste of the fruit complements the naturally sweet taste of the pork.

2 leeks, sliced

1 cup dried apricots

1 cup dried pears, sliced

½ cup golden raisins

1 (3-pound) boneless
   pork loin

½ teaspoon salt

1 teaspoon dried thyme leaves

1 cup apricot nectar

D Dairy-Free

G Gluten-Free

N Nut-Free

NUTRITION INFORMATION
Calories: 370; Carbohydrates: 38g;
Sugar: 10g; Fiber: 4g; Fat: 7g;
Saturated Fat: 2g; Protein: 40g;
Sodium: 239mg

1 In a 6-quart slow cooker, place the leeks, apricots, pears, and raisins. Top with the pork. Sprinkle the pork with the salt and thyme.

2 Pour the apricot nectar around the pork, over the fruit.

3 Cover and cook on low for 7 to 9 hours, or until the pork registers at least 150°F on a food thermometer.

INGREDIENT TIP
Many dried fruits are treated with sulfites as a preservative and have added sugars. When you buy dried fruit for this recipe, make sure that they are sulfur-free with no added sugar.

CURRIED PORK CHOPS

SERVES 8 // PREP TIME: 20 MINUTES // COOK TIME: 7 TO 8 HOURS

Curry powder is usually made with turmeric, a colorful spice that contains a compound called curcumin that may help prevent cancer. Enjoy this spicy recipe knowing that it's good for you!

2 onions, chopped

4 garlic cloves, minced

2 red bell peppers, stemmed, seeded, and chopped

2 yellow bell peppers, stemmed, seeded, and chopped

8 (5.5-ounce) bone-in pork loin chops

½ teaspoon salt

1 tablespoon curry powder

1 tablespoon grated fresh ginger root

1 cup Chicken Stock (page 26)

1   In a slow cooker, mix the onions, garlic, and bell peppers. Add the pork chops to the slow cooker, nestling them into the vegetables.

2   In a small bowl, mix the salt, curry powder, ginger root, and chicken stock, and pour into the slow cooker.

3   Cover and cook on low for 7 to 8 hours, or until the pork chops are very tender.

INGREDIENT TIP
You can make this recipe with boneless pork chops, but bone-in chops have more flavor and they will hold together better in the long, slow cooking time.

D Dairy-Free

G Gluten-Free

N Nut-Free

NUTRITION INFORMATION
Calorie: 306; Carbohydrates: 10g; Sugar: 3g; Fiber: 2g; Fat: 14g; Saturated Fat: 5g; Protein: 34g; Sodium: 268mg

STEAK DIANE

SERVES 8 // PREP TIME: 20 MINUTES // COOK TIME: 8 TO 10 HOURS

Steak Diane is a recipe typically made on the stove top with a really expensive cut of beef such as tenderloin, along with sautéed onions, mushrooms, and garlic. This slow cooker version is just as good, and it uses a more inexpensive cut.

2 onions, sliced

4 garlic cloves, sliced

2 shallots, peeled and sliced

2 cups sliced cremini mushrooms

5 large carrots, sliced

1 (3-pound) grass-fed chuck shoulder roast or tri-tip roast, cut into 2-inch pieces

2 tablespoons chopped fresh chives

1 teaspoon dried marjoram leaves

1 cup low-sodium beef broth

2 tablespoons butter

1 In a 6-quart slow cooker, mix the onions, garlic, shallots, mushrooms, and carrots.

2 Add the beef and stir gently. Sprinkle the chives and marjoram over the beef, and pour the beef broth over all.

3 Cover and cook on low for 8 to 10 hours, or until the beef is very tender.

4 Stir in the butter and serve.

SUBSTITUTION TIP
This recipe can also be made with pork loin. Just cut the pork into 2-inch pieces and add it to the slow cooker. Use chicken broth in place of the beef broth. The cooking time will be reduced to 6 to 8 hours.

G Gluten-Free

N Nut-Free

NUTRITION INFORMATION
Calories: 381; Carbohydrates: 11g;
Sugar: 5g; Fiber: 2g; Fat: 19g;
Saturated Fat: 8g; Protein: 38g;
Sodium: 162mg

ROAST PORK WITH CABBAGE

SERVES 8 // PREP TIME: 20 MINUTES // COOK TIME: 7 TO 9 HOURS

Pork cooked with cabbage is a classic combination often served in Germany. The sweet and sour cabbage is a perfect complement to the tender pork.

1 large head red cabbage, chopped

2 red onions, chopped

2 medium pears, peeled and chopped

4 garlic cloves, minced

1 cup Chicken Stock (page 26)

¼ cup apple cider vinegar

3 tablespoons honey

1 teaspoon dried thyme leaves

½ teaspoon salt

1 (3-pound) pork loin roast

Ⓓ Dairy-Free
Ⓖ Gluten-Free
Ⓝ Nut-Free

NUTRITION INFORMATION
Calories: 365; Carbohydrates: 21g; Sugar: 14g; Fiber: 3g; Fat: 14g; Saturated Fat: 3g; Protein: 38g; Sodium: 263mg

1   In a 6-quart slow cooker, mix the cabbage, onions, pears, and garlic.

2   In a small bowl, mix the chicken stock, vinegar, honey, thyme, and salt, and pour into the slow cooker.

3   Top with the pork, nestling the meat into the vegetables.

4   Cover and cook on low for 7 to 9 hours, or until the pork is tender.

RECIPE TIP
You can thicken the liquid in the slow cooker and turn it into gravy with any of these meat recipes by combining about 3 tablespoons cornstarch with ½ cup water or other liquid. Stir it into the slow cooker, then cover and cook on low for another 20 minutes or so until the liquid thickens.

THAI PORK WITH PEANUT SAUCE

SERVES 8 // PREP TIME: 20 MINUTES // COOK TIME: 7 TO 9 HOURS

Peanut sauce is a classic Thai recipe, made from peanut butter, soy sauce, garlic, vinegar, onions, and spices. Its richness complements the tender nuttiness of the pork in this easy recipe.

2 onions, chopped

2 cups chopped portabello mushrooms

4 garlic cloves, minced

1 small dried red chili pepper, sliced

¼ teaspoon cayenne pepper

1 cup peanut butter

1 cup Chicken Stock (page 26)

2 tablespoons apple cider vinegar

1 (3-pound) boneless pork loin roast

1 cup chopped unsalted peanuts

D Dairy-Free

G Gluten-Free

1 In a 6-quart slow cooker, mix the onions, mushrooms, garlic, chili pepper, and cayenne pepper.

2 In a medium bowl, mix the peanut butter, chicken stock, and vinegar and mix until well blended.

3 Place the pork roast in the slow cooker on top of the vegetables. Pour the peanut butter sauce over all.

4 Cover and cook on low for 7 to 9 hours, or until the pork is very tender.

5 Sprinkle with peanuts and serve.

INGREDIENT TIP
Peanut butter can be simply made, or it can be stuffed full of sugar and artificial ingredients. Read the label when you buy it, and purchase only peanut butter made with peanuts and salt.

NUTRITION INFORMATION
Calories: 664; Carbohydrates: 19g; Sugar: 6g; Fiber: 6g; Fat: 44g; Saturated Fat: 7g; Protein: 54g; Sodium: 232mg

LEMON-GARLIC PORK CHOPS

SERVES 8 // PREP TIME: 20 MINUTES // COOK TIME: 7 TO 8 HOURS

This recipe is similar to Shrimp Scampi (page 128), since lemon and garlic are the two main seasonings in that classic recipe. Serve this easy recipe over hot cooked brown rice for a great meal.

2 leeks, chopped

8 garlic cloves, sliced

2 red bell peppers, stemmed, seeded, and chopped

8 (5-ounce) bone-in pork loin chops

⅓ cup lemon juice

1 cup Chicken Stock (page 26)

1 teaspoon dried thyme leaves

½ teaspoon salt

1 In a 6-quart slow cooker, mix the leeks, garlic, and red bell peppers. Top with the pork chops.

2 In a small bowl, mix the lemon juice, chicken stock, thyme, and salt. Pour over the pork.

3 Cover and cook on low for 7 to 8 hours, or until the chops register at least 145°F on a food thermometer.

INGREDIENT TIP
Pork no longer has to be cooked well done, according to the USDA. Cook it until it registers 145°F. The pork can be slightly pink in the center and still be safe to eat.

D Dairy-Free

G Gluten-Free

N Nut-Free

NUTRITION INFORMATION
Calories: 269; Carbohydrates: 6g;
Sugar: 2g; Fiber: 1g; Fat: 13g;
Saturated Fat: 4g; Protein: 30g;
Sodium: 249mg

GARLIC-PARMESAN PORK

SERVES 8 // PREP TIME: 20 MINUTES // COOK TIME: 7 TO 9 HOURS

Pork is such a mild meat, and it pairs well with just about any flavor. Garlic and Parmesan cheese are the ingredients that make this recipe so delicious. This is a one-dish meal because carrots and potatoes are cooked along with the pork.

2 pounds small creamer potatoes, rinsed

4 large carrots, cut into chunks

1 onion, chopped

12 garlic cloves, divided

1 (3-pound) boneless pork loin

1 cup Chicken Stock (page 26)

1 teaspoon dried marjoram leaves

½ cup grated Parmesan cheese

G Gluten-Free

N Nut-Free

NUTRITION INFORMATION
Calories: 393; Carbohydrates: 27g; Sugar: 5g; Fiber: 3g; Fat: 11g; Saturated Fat: 4g; Protein: 45g; Sodium: 404mg

1 In a 6-quart slow cooker, mix the potatoes, carrots, and onions. Mince 6 of the garlic cloves and add them to the vegetables.

2 Cut the remaining 6 garlic cloves into slivers. With a sharp knife, poke holes in the pork loin and insert a garlic sliver into each hole.

3 Put the pork loin on the vegetables in the slow cooker.

4 Pour the chicken stock over all and sprinkle with the marjoram.

5 Cover and cook on low for 7 to 9 hours, or until the pork is tender.

6 Top with the Parmesan cheese and serve.

INGREDIENT TIP
If you use freshly grated Parmesan cheese, do not throw the rind away. Tuck it into soups and stews for great flavor. Or put it in next to the pork loin in this recipe.

THAI BEEF AND VEGGIES

SERVES 8 // PREP TIME: 20 MINUTES // COOK TIME: 8 TO 10 HOURS

Thai flavors are delicious with the rich flavor of beef. This recipe uses peanut butter, peanuts, coconut milk, and chili peppers for a spicy and smooth sauce that complements the beef and vegetables.

3 onions, chopped

6 garlic cloves, minced

3 large carrots, shredded

2 tablespoons grated fresh ginger root

3 large tomatoes, seeded and chopped

¾ cup peanut butter (see tip on page 148)

1 cup canned coconut milk

1 small red chili pepper, minced

3 tablespoons lime juice

½ cup Beef Stock (page 27)

2½ pounds grass-fed beef sirloin roast, cut into 2-inch pieces

Ⓓ Dairy-Free
Ⓖ Gluten-Free

NUTRITION INFORMATION
Calories: 530; Carbohydrates: 18g;
Sugar: 8g; Fiber: 5g; Fat: 35g;
Unsaturated Fat: 14g; Protein: 36g;
Sodium: 225mg

1 In a 6-quart slow cooker, mix the onions, garlic, carrots, ginger root, and tomatoes.

2 In a medium bowl, mix the peanut butter, coconut milk, chili pepper, lime juice, and beef stock until well blended.

3 Put the roast on top of the vegetables in the slow cooker and pour the peanut sauce over all.

4 Cover and cook on low for 8 to 10 hours, or until the beef is very tender.

VARIATION TIP
Other vegetables can be used in this fragrant recipe. Add a stalk of lemongrass (remove it and discard when the beef is done), or add some chopped red or orange bell peppers. Garnish with chopped peanuts if you'd like.

MOROCCAN BEEF TAGINE

SERVES 8 // PREP TIME: 20 MINUTES // COOK TIME: 8 TO 10 HOURS

Tagine is both the name of a dish and a pot in which the dish is cooked. The earthenware pot is topped with a conical lid that traps the heat and moisture as the food cooks—kind of like a slow cooker! This spicy recipe is perfect for entertaining.

2 onions, chopped

6 garlic cloves, minced

2 jalapeño peppers, minced

3 carrots, cut into chunks

1 cup chopped dates

1 (3-pound) grass-fed beef sirloin roast, cut into 2-inch pieces

2 tablespoons honey

1 cup Beef Stock (page 27)

2 teaspoons ground cumin

1 teaspoon ground turmeric

(D) Dairy-Free

(G) Gluten-Free

(N) Nut-Free

1 In a 6-quart slow cooker, mix the onions, garlic, jalapeño peppers, carrots, and dates. Top with the beef.

2 In a small bowl, mix the honey, beef stock, cumin, and turmeric until well combined. Pour into the slow cooker.

3 Cover and cook on low for 8 to 10 hours, or until the beef is very tender.

INGREDIENT TIP
Dates may seem like dried fruit, but they are really fresh fruit. The best kind is called "Medjool." Dates are rich and thick and add a honey-like flavor to this recipe. They are high in B vitamins and potassium, along with vitamins A and K.

NUTRITION INFORMATION
Calories: 452; Carbohydrates: 29g; Sugar: 22g; Fiber: 4g; Fat: 21g; Saturated Fat: 9g; Protein: 35g; Sodium: 154mg

MOROCCAN BEEF IN LETTUCE CUPS

SERVES 8 // PREP TIME: 20 MINUTES // COOK TIME: 7 TO 9 HOURS

Moroccan food is very fragrant, since the cuisine uses warm spices to season recipes. Cumin, cinnamon, and garlic are the most commonly used flavorings. This fun recipe cooks beef until it is meltingly tender. You then serve the beef in lettuce cups and top it with pomegranate seeds, spicy radishes, and grated carrot.

4 garlic cloves, cut into slivers

3 pounds grass-fed beef sirloin roast

½ cup Beef Stock (page 27)

1 (14-ounce) BPA-free can no-salt-added diced tomatoes, undrained

¼ cup tomato paste (see tip on page 31)

1 teaspoon ground cumin

1 teaspoon ground cinnamon

½ cup pomegranate seeds

4 radishes, thinly sliced

1 cup grated carrot

20 butter lettuce leaves

D Dairy-Free

G Gluten-Free

N Nut-Free

1 Poke holes in the sirloin roast and insert the slivers of garlic. Put the roast into a 6-quart slow cooker.

2 In a medium bowl, mix the beef stock, tomatoes, tomato paste, cumin, and cinnamon until well blended. Pour over the roast.

3 Cover and cook on low for 7 to 9 hours or until the beef is very tender.

4 Remove the beef from the slow cooker and shred using two forks. Combine the beef with about 1 cup of the liquid from the slow cooker in a large serving bowl.

5 Serve the beef mixture with the remaining ingredients and let each diner assemble their meal.

INGREDIENT TIP

To remove the seeds from pomegranates, cut each in half. Then use a wooden spoon or a rolling pin to hit the pomegranate half. The seeds will come out easily. You can sometimes buy pomegranate seeds in the produce aisle of large supermarkets.

NUTRITION INFORMATION

Calories: 376; Carbohydrates: 9g; Sugar: 5g; Fiber: 2g; Fat: 21g; Saturated Fat: 9g; Protein: 35g; Sodium: 141mg

BEEF BRISKET BBQ

SERVES 8 // PREP TIME: 20 MINUTES // COOK TIME: 8 TO 11 HOURS

Purchased barbecue sauces are full of ingredients such as high fructose corn syrup, sugar, and artificial colors. It's easy to make your own barbecue by first rubbing the meat with spices, then cooking it in a spicy tomato sauce.

3 onions, chopped

8 garlic cloves, minced

2 teaspoons paprika

1 teaspoon dried oregano leaves

1 teaspoon dried marjoram leaves

½ teaspoon cayenne pepper

1 (3-pound) grass-fed beef brisket, trimmed

2 (8-ounce) BPA-free cans no-salt-added tomato sauce

⅓ cup natural mustard

3 tablespoons honey

Ⓓ Dairy-Free
Ⓖ Gluten-Free
Ⓝ Nut-Free

NUTRITION INFORMATION
Calories: 303; Carbohydrates: 18g; Sugar: 12g; Fiber: 2g; Fat: 10g; Saturated Fat: 3g; Protein: 37g; Sodium: 277mg

1 In a 6-quart slow cooker, mix the onions and garlic.

2 In a small bowl, mix the paprika, oregano, marjoram, and cayenne. Rub this mixture into the beef brisket.

3 In another small bowl, mix the tomato sauce, mustard, and honey until well combined.

4 Put the beef on the onions and garlic in the slow cooker. Pour the tomato mixture over all.

5 Cover and cook on low for 8 to 11 hours, or until the beef is very tender.

6 You can slice the beef to serve it or shred it to serve on buns.

INGREDIENT TIP
Brisket is a specific cut of meat from the lower chest, one of the nine primal cuts. It is rich and tender when slowly cooked. The collagen in the meat gelatinizes as it cooks, which acts as a self-marinade.

BEEF LO MEIN

SERVES 8 // PREP TIME: 20 MINUTES // COOK TIME: 8½ TO 10½ HOURS

Lo mein just means meat and vegetables served with wheat noodles. The beef becomes very tender and almost velvety when cooked this way. And the pasta cooks right in the sauce, which means it is more flavorful than pasta cooked in water.

2 onions, chopped

2 cups shiitake mushrooms, sliced

4 garlic cloves, minced

1 tablespoon grated fresh ginger root

1 jalapeño pepper, minced

2 pounds grass-fed beef chuck roast, cut into 2-inch pieces

3 cups Beef Stock (page 27)

2 tablespoons low-sodium soy sauce

2 tablespoons honey

1 (8-ounce) package whole-wheat spaghetti pasta, broken in half

Ⓓ Dairy-Free

Ⓝ Nut-Free

NUTRITION INFORMATION
Calories: 355; Carbohydrates: 33g; Sugar: 8g; Fiber: 4g; Fat: 14g; Saturated Fat: 5g; Protein: 28g; Sodium: 294mg

1 In a 6-quart slow cooker, mix the onions, mushrooms, garlic, ginger root, and jalapeño pepper. Add the beef cubes and stir.

2 In a medium bowl, mix the beef stock, soy sauce, and honey until well combined. Pour into the slow cooker.

3 Cover and cook on low for 8 to 10 hours, or until the beef is very tender.

4 Turn the slow cooker to high heat. Add the pasta and stir gently, making sure all of the spaghetti is covered with liquid.

5 Cook on high for 20 to 30 minutes, or until the pasta is tender.

RECIPE TIP
This recipe is so much better and so much better for you than Chinese takeout! Add more veggies to it to make it healthier. Some grated carrots, chopped bell peppers, and green beans would be delicious additions.

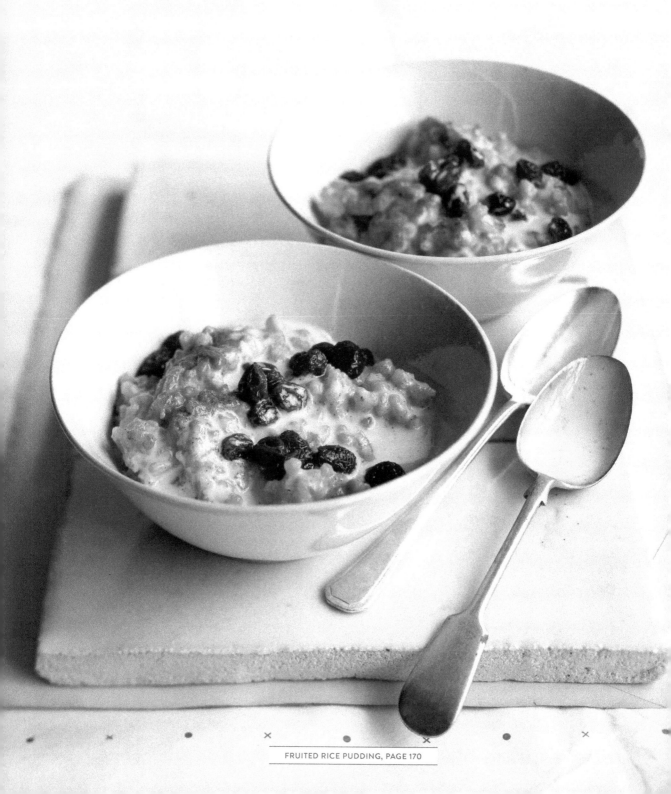

FRUITED RICE PUDDING, PAGE 170

CHAPTER TEN

APPS AND SWEETS

APPLE-PEACH CRUMBLE

SERVES 8 // PREP TIME: 20 MINUTES // COOK TIME: 4 TO 5 HOURS

Apple crumble is made of a combination of apples, peaches, and a sweet oatmeal mixture that becomes rich and almost candy-like as it cooks. Enjoy this dish with some frozen yogurt for a great dessert.

6 large Granny Smith apples, peeled and cut into chunks

4 large peaches, peeled and sliced

3 tablespoons honey

2 tablespoons lemon juice

1 cup almond flour

1 teaspoon ground cinnamon

3 cups quick-cooking oatmeal

⅓ cup coconut sugar

½ cup slivered almonds

½ cup coconut oil, melted

D Dairy-Free
G Gluten-Free
V Vegetarian

NUTRITION INFORMATION
Calories: 547; Carbohydrates: 75g; Sugar: 42g; Fiber: 11g; Fat: 26g; Saturated Fat: 14g; Protein: 10g; Sodium: 0g

1 In a 6-quart slow cooker, mix the apples, peaches, honey, and lemon juice.

2 In a large bowl, mix the almond flour, cinnamon, oatmeal, coconut sugar, and almonds until well combined.

3 Add the coconut oil and mix until crumbly.

4 Sprinkle the almond mixture over the fruit in the slow cooker.

5 Cover and cook on low for 4 to 5 hours, or until the fruit is tender and the crumble is bubbling around the edges.

INGREDIENT TIP
Granny Smith apples have a wonderful tart flavor, and they brown less quickly than other varieties after they are cut. They are easy to find in any grocery store.

BERRY CRISP

SERVES 12 // PREP TIME: 20 MINUTES // COOK TIME: 5 TO 6 HOURS

Frozen berries are the perfect choice for making this dessert in the slow cooker. They keep their shape better than fresh fruit during the long cooking time. Look for organic versions in the frozen food aisle.

3 cups frozen organic blueberries

3 cups frozen organic raspberries

3 cups frozen organic strawberries

2 tablespoons lemon juice

2½ cups rolled oats

1 cup whole-wheat flour

⅓ cup maple sugar

1 teaspoon ground cinnamon

⅓ cup coconut oil, melted

Ⓓ Dairy-Free

Ⓥ Vegan

NUTRITION INFORMATION
Calories: 219; Carbohydrates: 37g; Sugar: 12g; Fiber: 7g; Fat: 8g; Saturated Fat: 5g; Protein: 5g; Sodium: 9mg

1 Do not thaw the berries. In a 6-quart slow cooker, mix the frozen berries. Drizzle with the lemon juice.

2 In a large bowl, mix the oats, flour, maple sugar, and cinnamon until well combined. Stir in the melted coconut oil until crumbly.

3 Sprinkle the oat mixture over the fruit in the slow cooker.

4 Cover and cook on low for 5 to 6 hours, or until the fruit is bubbling and the topping is browned.

INGREDIENT TIP
Maple sugar is made from pure maple syrup. The syrup is boiled until it starts to "sugar," that is, grains appear in the syrup. It is a pure sweetener and is approved for the eating clean plan.

PEACH BROWN BETTY

SERVES 10 // PREP TIME: 20 MINUTES // COOK TIME: 5 TO 6 HOURS

"Brown Betty" is an old-fashioned dessert made with fruit topped with sweetened bread cubes or crumbs. You can make the bread yourself, or buy it at the store. Be sure to read the label and buy only bread made with ingredients you would use at home.

8 ripe peaches, peeled and cut into chunks

1 cup dried cranberries (see tip on page 68)

2 tablespoons freshly squeezed lemon juice

3 tablespoons honey

3 cups cubed whole-wheat bread (see tip on page 57)

1½ cups whole-wheat bread crumbs

⅓ cup coconut sugar

¼ teaspoon ground cardamom

⅓ cup melted coconut oil

1 In a 6-quart slow cooker, mix the peaches, dried cranberries, lemon juice, and honey.

2 In a large bowl, mix the bread cubes, bread crumbs, coconut sugar, and cardamom. Drizzle the melted coconut oil over all and toss to coat.

3 Sprinkle the bread mixture on the fruit in the slow cooker.

4 Cover and cook on low for 5 to 6 hours, or until the fruit is bubbling and the topping is browned.

INGREDIENT TIP
Coconut sugar looks like brown sugar, but it doesn't pack into a measuring cup. It has a rich flavor and contains nutrients such as iron, zinc, calcium, and potassium. This sugar also has a fiber called inulin, which can slow glucose absorption in your body.

Ⓓ Dairy-Free

Ⓥ Vegetarian

NUTRITION INFORMATION
Calories: 322; Carbohydrates: 57g; Sugar: 31g; Fiber: 6g; Fat: 9g; Saturated Fat: 7g; Protein: 6g; Sodium: 69mg

NUTTY BAKED APPLES

SERVES 8 // PREP TIME: 20 MINUTES // COOK TIME: 4 TO 6 HOURS

Apples are cored and stuffed with a sweetened nut filling in this old-fashioned and classic recipe. Choose large and firm apples that will stand up to long cooking times.

8 large apples

2 tablespoons freshly squeezed lemon juice

1½ cups buckwheat flakes

1 cup chopped walnuts

⅓ cup coconut sugar

1 teaspoon ground cinnamon

¼ teaspoon salt

6 tablespoons unsalted butter, cut into pieces

½ cup apple juice

Ⓖ Gluten-Free

Ⓥ Vegetarian

NUTRITION INFORMATION
Calories: 369; Carbohydrates: 53g;
Sugar: 36g; Fiber: 6g; Fat: 17g;
Saturated Fat: 6g; Protein: 4g;
Sodium: 112mg

1 Peel a strip of skin around the top of each apple to prevent splitting. Carefully remove the apple core, making sure not to cut all the way through to the bottom. Brush the apples with lemon juice and set aside.

2 In a medium bowl, mix the buckwheat flakes, walnuts, coconut sugar, cinnamon, and salt.

3 Drizzle the melted butter over the buckwheat mixture and mix until crumbly. Use this mixture to stuff the apples, rounding the stuffing on top of each apple.

4 In a 6-quart slow cooker, place the stuffed apples. Pour the apple juice around the apples.

5 Cover and cook on low for 4 to 6 hours, or until the apples are very tender.

INGREDIENT TIP
The best apples for baking and cooking are Granny Smith, Jonagold, Jonathan, McIntosh, Crispin, Winesap, Fuji, Honeycrisp, and Cortland. They hold their shape after they are cooked.

SPICED CARROT PUDDING

SERVES 12 // PREP TIME: 20 MINUTES // COOK TIME: 5 TO 7 HOURS

A pudding like this one is usually steamed. But the slow cooker is a great substitute for a steamer. Make sure that you grate the carrots using the smallest holes on your grater. This recipe is comforting and mild and sweet, perfect for a cold winter night.

3 cups finely grated carrots

1½ cups chopped pecans

1 cup golden raisins

1 cup almond flour

1 cup coconut flour

½ cup coconut sugar

1 teaspoon baking powder

1½ teaspoons ground cinnamon

2 eggs, beaten

2 cups canned coconut milk

1 In a 6-quart slow cooker, mix all of the ingredients. Cover and cook on low for 5 to 7 hours, or until the pudding is set.

2 Serve warm, either plain or with softly whipped heavy cream.

INGREDIENT TIP
Almond flour and coconut flour are two gluten-free flours that have a mild taste and good texture. You could use 2 cups of all-purpose flour or whole-wheat pastry flour in place of the gluten-free flours if you'd like.

Ⓓ Dairy-Free
Ⓖ Gluten-Free
Ⓥ Vegetarian

NUTRITION INFORMATION
Calories: 359; Carbohydrates: 31g; Sugar: 22g; Fiber: 7g; Fat: 24g; Saturated Fat: 10g; Protein: 7g; Sodium: 70mg

SPINACH AND ARTICHOKE DIP

SERVES 10 // PREP TIME: 20 MINUTES // COOK TIME: 4 TO 5 HOURS

This is a eating clean version of the popular warm dip often found in restaurants. That version is made with mayonnaise and lots of different kinds of cheese. Mashed cannellini beans stand in for most of the mayonnaise and cheese. Serve with toasted bread and crudités.

1 (15-ounce) BPA-free can no-salt-added cannellini beans, drained and rinsed

1 red onion, chopped

3 garlic cloves, minced

2 (14-ounce) BPA-free cans no-salt-added artichoke hearts, drained and quartered

1 (10-ounce) bag chopped frozen spinach, thawed and drained

½ cup sour cream

2 tablespoons freshly squeezed lemon juice

2 tablespoons olive oil

1 cup shredded Swiss cheese

1 In a 6-quart slow cooker, mash the beans using a potato masher.

2 Stir in the onion, garlic, and artichoke hearts.

3 Stir in the spinach, sour cream, lemon juice, olive oil, and Swiss cheese.

4 Cover and cook on low for 4 to 5 hours, or until the dip is hot and bubbling.

SUBSTITUTION TIP
You can substitute any chopped fresh leafy green for the frozen spinach if you'd like. Use 2 cups chopped kale, collard greens, or mustard greens.

G Gluten-Free

N Nut-Free

V Vegetarian

NUTRITION INFORMATION
Calories: 145; Carbohydrates: 10g;
Sugar: 1g; Fiber: 4g; Fat: 9g;
Saturated Fat: 4g; Protein: 6g;
Sodium: 54mg

TEX-MEX NACHO DIP

SERVES 12 // PREP TIME: 20 MINUTES // COOK TIME: 6 TO 8 HOURS

Nachos are typically made with beef and some type of plastic cheese, cooked until hot, then poured over tortilla chips and broiled. This dip has all the flavors of the original but is much healthier because it is made with chicken and Greek yogurt. Serve with tortilla chips and crudités.

4 (5-ounce) boneless, skinless chicken breasts

3 onions, chopped

6 garlic cloves, minced

2 jalapeño peppers, minced

½ cup Chicken Stock (page 26)

2 tablespoons chili powder

1 (15-ounce) BPA-free can no-salt-added black beans, drained and rinsed

1 cup plain Greek yogurt

1 cup shredded Monterey Jack cheese

2 avocados, peeled and chopped

1 In a 6-quart slow cooker, mix the chicken, onions, garlic, and jalapeño peppers. Add the chicken stock and chili powder. Cover and cook on low for 5 to 7 hours, or until the chicken registers 165°F on a food thermometer.

2 Remove the chicken from the slow cooker and shred it using two forks. Return the chicken to the slow cooker.

3 Add the black beans, yogurt, and cheese. Cover and cook on low 1 hour longer, until hot.

4 Top with the avocados and serve.

VARIATION TIP
This recipe makes a great soup if you just add more chicken stock. Add 4 cups when you cook the chicken. Also add 2 tablespoons cornstarch stirred into the Greek yogurt to thicken the soup slightly.

Ⓖ Gluten-Free

Ⓝ Nut-Free

NUTRITION INFORMATION
Calories: 218; Carbohydrates: 13g;
Sugar: 4g; Fiber: 4g; Fat: 11g;
Saturated Fat: 5g; Protein: 18g;
Sodium: 286mg

SPICED CHOCOLATE-NUT CLUSTERS

Candy made in the slow cooker always amazes people. The slow cooker is really used as a chocolate melter in this recipe. You can make a ton of candies this way; give them for Christmas gifts!

4 pounds dairy-free 70% to 80% cacao dark chocolate, chopped

¼ cup coconut oil

2 teaspoons vanilla extract

1 teaspoon ground cinnamon

¼ teaspoon ground cloves

4 cups roasted cashews

3 cups coarsely chopped pecans

D Dairy-Free

G Gluten-Free

V Vegetarian

NUTRITION INFORMATION
Calories: 271; Carbohydrates: 17g; Sugar: 8g; Fiber: 4g; Fat: 21g; Saturated Fat: 9g; Protein: 4g; Sodium: 6mg

1 In a 6-quart slow cooker, mix the chopped chocolate, coconut oil, vanilla, cinnamon, and cloves. Cover and cook on low for 2 hours, or until the chocolate melts.

2 Stir the chocolate mixture until it is smooth.

3 Stir in the cashews and pecans.

4 Drop the mixture by tablespoons onto waxed paper or parchment paper. Let stand until set.

INGREDIENT TIP
The healthiest chocolate has at least 70 percent cacao. This type of chocolate has fiber, iron, magnesium, potassium, and zinc, and it has lots of healthy antioxidants.

APPLE-OATMEAL BREAD PUDDING

SERVES 8 // PREP TIME: 20 MINUTES // COOK TIME: 6 TO 8 HOURS

Bread pudding is a classic old-fashioned recipe that is pure comfort food. Unfortunately, it is usually made with white bread and packed with sugar. This updated recipe is good for you and very flavorful.

8 slices oatmeal bread, cubed

2 cups quick-cooking oatmeal

3 apples, peeled and chopped

1 cup dried cranberries (see tip on page 68)

⅓ cup coconut sugar

1 teaspoon ground cinnamon

2 teaspoons vanilla extract

3 eggs, beaten

2 cups canned coconut milk

3 tablespoons coconut oil, melted

1 In a 6-quart slow cooker, mix the bread cubes, oatmeal, apples, and cranberries.

2 In a large bowl, mix the coconut sugar, cinnamon, vanilla, eggs, coconut milk, and melted coconut oil, and mix until well combined. Pour into the slow cooker.

3 Cover and cook on low for 6 to 8 hours, or until a food thermometer registers 165°F.

RECIPE TIP
Serve this bread pudding warm, with some frozen yogurt on top. It's great for breakfast or a snack as well as dessert.

D Dairy-Free

V Vegetarian

NUTRITION INFORMATION
Calories: 491; Carbohydrates: 69g; Sugar: 32g; Fiber: 9g; Fat: 21g; Saturated Fat: 17g; Protein: 10g; Sodium: 147mg

MOLE CHICKEN BITES

SERVES 8 // PREP TIME: 20 MINUTES // COOK TIME: 4 TO 6 HOURS

Most slow cooker chicken appetizer recipes are made with chicken wings, which have very little meat and are higher in fat. This appetizer recipe is made with chicken strips, which provide more protein. "Mole" is a Mexican recipe made with lots of chilies and cocoa powder, which adds a rich depth of flavor.

2 onions, chopped

6 garlic cloves, minced

4 large tomatoes, seeded and chopped

2 dried red chilies, crushed

1 jalapeño pepper, minced

2 tablespoons chili powder

3 tablespoons cocoa powder

2 tablespoons coconut sugar

½ cup Chicken Stock (page 26)

6 (5-ounce) boneless, skinless chicken breasts

Ⓓ Dairy-Free
Ⓖ Gluten-Free

1 In a 6-quart slow cooker, mix the onions, garlic, tomatoes, chili peppers, and jalapeño peppers.

2 In a medium bowl, mix the chili powder, cocoa powder, coconut sugar, and chicken stock.

3 Cut the chicken breasts into 1-inch strips crosswise and add to the slow cooker. Pour the chicken stock mixture over all.

4 Cover and cook on low for 4 to 6 hours, or until the chicken registers 165°F on a food thermometer. Serve with toothpicks or little plates and forks.

INGREDIENT TIP
Cocoa powder contains no sugar; it is made from dried, roasted, and ground cocoa beans with the fat removed. It contains iron, manganese, zinc, and magnesium along with flavonoids that act as antioxidants.

NUTRITION INFORMATION
Calories: 157; Carbohydrates: 12g;
Sugar: 8g; Fiber: 2g; Fat: 3g;
Saturated Fat: 0g; Protein: 23g;
Sodium: 249mg

SPICED NUT MIX

MAKES 12 CUPS // PREP TIME: 20 MINUTES // COOK TIME: 2 TO 3 HOURS

The slow cooker roasts nuts to golden perfection. You can make this recipe as spicy or as mild as you'd like. It's great for holiday parties or to give as gifts.

3 cups raw cashews

3 cups walnuts

3 cups pecans

3 cups macadamia nuts

¼ cup unsalted
   butter, melted

½ cup coconut sugar

2 tablespoons chili powder

2 teaspoons paprika

¼ teaspoon cayenne pepper

G Gluten-Free

V Vegetarian

NUTRITION INFORMATION
(PER ½ CUP SERVING)
Calories: 393; Carbohydrates: 10g;
Sugar: 2g; Fiber: 4g; Fat: 38g;
Saturated Fat: 6g; Protein: 7g;
Sodium: 60mg

1 In a 6-quart slow cooker, mix the cashews, walnuts, pecans, and macadamia nuts. Drizzle with the melted butter and toss.

2 In a small bowl, mix the coconut sugar, chili powder, paprika, and cayenne pepper until well combined. Sprinkle over the nuts and toss.

3 Partially cover the slow cooker and cook on low for 2 to 3 hours, stirring twice during cooking time, until the nuts are golden and toasted.

VARIATION TIP
Other nuts can be used in this recipe. You can use whole peanuts, hazelnuts, almonds, or pistachios. Just make sure that they add up to 12 cups.

CARAMELIZED ONION DIP

SERVES 12 // PREP TIME: 20 MINUTES // COOK TIME: 8 ½ TO 10 ½ HOURS

Everyone has had the ubiquitous onion dip made with a soup mix and sour cream. This appetizer recipe is different. Onions are caramelized in the slow cooker until they are sweet and tender, then mixed with Greek yogurt and lots of seasonings.

2 white onions, chopped

3 onions, sliced

2 cups sliced cremini mushrooms

6 garlic cloves, minced

2 tablespoons unsalted butter

1 bay leaf

1 teaspoon dried thyme leaves

2 tablespoons balsamic vinegar

2 ½ cups grated Gruyère cheese

2 tablespoons cornstarch

Ⓖ Gluten-Free

Ⓝ Nut-Free

Ⓥ Vegetarian

NUTRITION INFORMATION
Calories: 263; Carbohydrates: 9g; Sugar: 4g; Fiber: 1g; Fat: 17g; Saturated Fat: 11g; Protein: 15g; Sodium: 386mg

1 In a 6-quart slow cooker, mix the onions, mushrooms, garlic, butter, bay leaf, thyme, and balsamic vinegar.

2 Cover and cook on low for 8 to 10 hours, or until the onions are deep golden brown and very soft. Remove and discard the bay leaf.

3 Toss the cheese with the cornstarch in a medium bowl and then add to the slow cooker.

4 Cover and cook on low for another 20 to 30 minutes, or until the cheese has melted.

5 Serve with crudités and tortilla chips.

INGREDIENT TIP
Gruyère cheese is a type of Swiss cheese that has a stronger and richer taste. You can find it in most large grocery stores. If you can't buy Gruyère, Swiss makes a good substitute.

FRUITED RICE PUDDING

SERVES 16 // PREP TIME: 20 MINUTES // COOK TIME: 5 TO 6 HOURS

Rice pudding is pure comfort food. This recipe is made with short-grain brown rice, which releases starch as it cooks for hours. The pudding is very creamy and fragrant. It is topped with toasted nuts and, if you like, some dark chocolate chips for an indulgent touch.

6 cups canned coconut milk

3 cups water

1⅔ cups brown Arborio rice

½ cup coconut sugar

2 tablespoons coconut oil

1 cup raisins

1 tablespoon vanilla extract

1 cup dark chocolate chips (optional)

G Gluten-Free

V Vegan

NUTRITION INFORMATION
Calories: 383; Carbohydrates: 41g;
Sugar: 22g; Fiber: 2g; Fat: 24g;
Saturated Fat: 21g; Protein: 5g;
Sodium: 27mg

1 In a 6-quart slow cooker, mix the coconut milk and water. Add the rice and coconut sugar and mix. Add the coconut oil and the raisins.

2 Cover and cook on low for 5 to 6 hours, or until the rice is very tender.

3 Stir in the vanilla. If using, serve the pudding with the chocolate chips sprinkled on top.

INGREDIENT TIP
Brown Arborio rice can be difficult to find. If you can't find it in your supermarket, you can substitute any short-grain brown rice. You can also use medium grain rice, but the pudding won't be quite as creamy.

CLEAN EATING BROWNIES

SERVES 12 // PREP TIME: 20 MINUTES // COOK TIME: 4 TO 5 HOURS

Believe it or not, you can make brownies in a slow cooker! And because this cooking method is gentle and moist, the brownies will be incredibly fudgy and creamy. Using pureed pears and some mashed bananas in this recipe adds nutrition and helps reduce the fat content.

1½ cups whole-wheat pastry flour

¾ cup unsweetened cocoa powder

1 teaspoon baking powder

5 tablespoons coconut oil, melted

1 cup mashed ripe bananas (about 2 medium)

1 cup mashed peeled ripe pears

½ cup coconut sugar

½ cup honey

4 eggs

2 teaspoons vanilla extract

Ⓓ Dairy-Free

NUTRITION INFORMATION
Calories: 260; Carbohydrates: 43g; Sugar: 25g; Fiber: 5g; Fat: 8g; Saturated fat: 6g; Protein: 2g; Sodium: 47mg

1 Tear off two long strips of heavy-duty foil and fold to make long thin strips. Place in a 6-quart slow cooker to make an X. Then line the slow cooker with parchment paper on top of the foil.

2 In a medium bowl, combine the whole-wheat pastry flour, cocoa powder, and baking powder and stir to mix.

3 In another medium bowl, combine the melted coconut oil, mashed bananas, mashed pears, coconut sugar, honey, eggs, and vanilla and mix well.

4 Stir the banana mixture into the flour mixture just until combined.

5 Spoon the batter into the slow cooker onto the parchment paper.

6 Cover and cook on low for 4 to 5 hours or until a toothpick inserted near the center comes out with just a few moist crumbs attached to it.

7 Carefully remove the brownie, using the foil sling. Let cool, then remove the brownie from the parchment paper and cut into squares to serve.

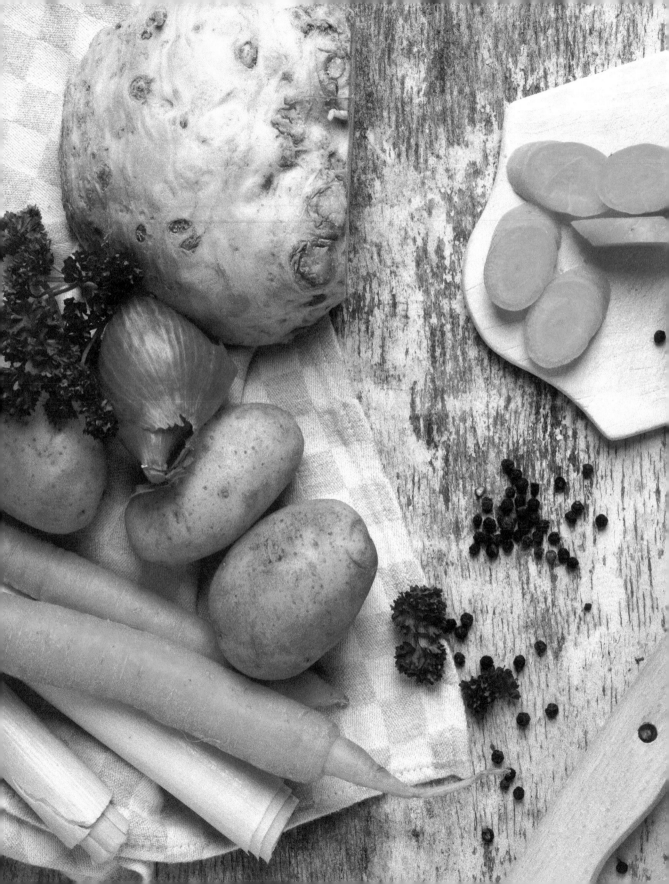

the dirty dozen and the clean fifteen

A nonprofit and environmental watchdog organization called the Environmental Working Group (EWG) looks at data supplied by the US Department of Agriculture (USDA) and the Food and Drug Administration (FDA) about pesticide residues. Each year, it compiles a list of the lowest and highest pesticide loads found in commercial crops. You can use these lists to decide which fruits and vegetables to buy organic to minimize your exposure to pesticides and which conventional produce is considered safe enough to eat. This does not mean they are pesticide-free, though, so wash these (and all) fruits and vegetables thoroughly.

These lists change every year, so make sure you look up the most recent one before you fill your shopping cart. You'll find the most recent lists as well as a guide to pesticides in produce at EWG.org/FoodNews.

THE DIRTY DOZEN

Apples · Celery · Cherry tomatoes · Cucumbers · Grapes
Nectarines (imported) · Peaches · Potatoes · Snap peas (imported)
Spinach · Strawberries · Sweet bell peppers
(Kale/Collard greens · Hot peppers)

** In addition to the dirty dozen, the EWG added two produce items contaminated with highly toxic organophosphate insecticides.

THE CLEAN FIFTEEN

Asparagus · Avocados · Cabbage · Cantaloupes (domestic)
Cauliflower · Eggplant · Grapefruit · Kiwifruit
Mangos · Onions · Papayas · Pineapples · Sweet corn
Sweet peas (frozen) · Sweet potatoes

Measurement Conversions

VOLUME EQUIVALENTS (LIQUID)

US STANDARD (OUNCES)	US STANDARD (APPROXIMATE)	METRIC
2 tablespoons	1 fl. oz.	30 mL
¼ cup	2 fl. oz.	60 mL
½ cup	4 fl. oz.	120 mL
1 cup	8 fl. oz.	240 mL
1½ cups	12 fl. oz.	355 mL
2 cups or 1 pint	16 fl. oz.	475 mL
4 cups or 1 quart	32 fl. oz.	1 L
1 gallon	128 fl. oz.	4 L

OVEN TEMPERATURE

FAHRENHEIT (F)	CELSIUS (C) (APPROXIMATE)
250°F	120°C
300°F	150°C
325°F	165°C
350°F	180°C
375°F	190°C
400°F	200°C
425°F	220°C
450°F	230°C

VOLUME EQUIVALENTS (DRY)

US STANDARD	METRIC (APPROXIMATE)
¼ teaspoon	1 mL
½ teaspoon	2 mL
1 teaspoon	5 mL
1 tablespoon	15 mL
¼ cup	59 mL
⅓ cup	79 mL
½ cup	118 mL
1 cup	177 mL

WEIGHT EQUIVALENTS

US STANDARD	METRIC (APPROXIMATE)
½ ounce	15 g
1 ounce	30 g
2 ounces	60 g
4 ounces	115 g
8 ounces	225 g
12 ounces	340 g
16 ounces or 1 pound	455 g

Resources

SLOW COOKER MANUALS

Most manuals for slow cookers can be downloaded from the Web. It can be helpful to download manuals for slow cookers other than the one you purchased, just for more ideas, recipes, and tips.

CROCK-POT: Manuals for Crock-Pot brand slow cookers can be found at www.crock-pot.com/service-and-support/product-support/instruction-manuals/instruction-manuals.html, and they usually include a user manual, quick start guide, and recipe booklet.

WEST BEND: West Bend slow cooker manuals can be found at www.westbend.com/support/user-manuals/slow-cookers.html. Cooking tips and some good recipes are included.

HAMILTON BEACH: Manuals for Hamilton Beach slow cookers are found at https://www.manualslib.com/brand/hamilton-beach/slow-cooker.html. The site also offers recipes.

WEBSITES FOR HEALTHY RECIPES

Some websites have tasty and easy healthy recipes for the slow cooker. Unfortunately, many slow cooker recipes use foods such as canned condensed soups and convenience foods that are high in sodium, fat, and artificial ingredients. The recipes on the following sites, however, are good for you.

EATING WELL has some great recipes, including ones for French Onion Soup and Pulled Pork. Find them at www.eatingwell.com/recipes/17987/cooking-methods/slow-cooker-crockpot/

TASTE OF HOME offers delicious and comforting healthy slow cooker recipes, including Sunday Pot Roast, Seafood Cioppino, and Beans 'n' Pumpkin Chili. www.tasteofhome.com/recipes/healthy-eating/healthy-slow-cooker-recipes

CLEAN EATING RECIPES has a section devoted to the slow cooker. Some dishes include Whole-Wheat Crockpot Pot Bread, Molten Lava Cake, and Chili Verde. www.cleaneatingrecipes.com/clean-eating-crock-pot-recipes/.

CLEAN EATING MAGAZINE has an online presence too. This page offers seven days of clean eating slow cooker recipes: www.cleaneatingmag.com/slideshow /7-days-of-slow-cooker-recipes/.

ANDREA'S NOTEBOOK has 150 clean eating slow cooker recipes that sound delicious. www.andreasnotebook.com/clean-eating-crock-pot-recipes/.

BOOKS AND WEBSITES FOR CLEAN EATING

Books and websites dedicated to clean eating offer lots of tips to adapt to the lifestyle, along with some great recipes.

PREVENTION MAGAZINE has lots of information about clean eating. You can find great recipes for foods such as Squachos, Energy Bars, and Butternut Squash Winter Salad. www.prevention.com/eatclean.

THE GRACIOUS PANTRY offers some delicious recipes including Taco Soup, Pineapple Chicken Verde, and Spaghetti Meatball Sandwiches. www.thegraciouspantry.com/category/recipes/slow-cooker-recipes/.

Clean Eating: Top Slow Cooker Recipes is a book that offers more than 230 recipes for the slow cooker. www.amazon.com/Clean-Eating-Recipes-Delicious -Cookbook/dp /1536990957/ref=sr_1_1?ie=UTF8&qid=1484768446&sr=8-1.

Eating Clean: The 21-Day Plan to Detox, Fight Inflammation, and Reset Your Body offers some great tips and delicious recipes for jumping into the clean eating plan. www.amazon.com/Eating-Clean-21-Day-Detox-Inflammation /dp/0544546466/ref =sr_1_4?ie=UTF8&qid=1484768499&sr=8-4.

The second edition of *Eating Clean for Dummies*, written by Linda Larsen and Dr. Jonathan Wright, offers a very detailed look into the science and chemistry behind the clean eating plan. And we include a few recipes. www.amazon .com/Eating-Clean-Dummies-Jonathan-Wright/dp/1119272211/ref=sr_1_1?ie =UTF8&qid=1484768563&sr=8-1.

Recipe Index

Index

N

Nut-free

About the Author

Linda Larsen is a journalist and home economist. She has a degree in Biology from St. Olaf College and a degree with High Distinction in Food Science and Nutrition from the University of Minnesota. She has been the Expert for Busy Cooks for About.com since 2002. She worked for the Pillsbury Company on the Bake-Off and in their test kitchens from 1988 to 2014. Linda has written 37 cookbooks since 2005, including *The Complete Slow Cooking for Two*, the *Ultimate Vegetarian Slow Cooker*, and *Eating Clean for Dummies*.

CPSIA information can be obtained
at www.ICGtesting.com
Printed in the USA
LVHW01s1407211217
560373LV00001B/1/P

9 781623 159108